Michael Lipman was born in England and raised in Sydney. He represented Australia in rugby union at under-19 level as a flanker before playing for the England national team. Michael played professionally in both England and Australia for Bristol, Bath and the Melbourne Rebels. In 2020 Michael was diagnosed with probable CTE and early-onset dementia. His goal is to change concussion protocols in contact sports.

Frankie Lipman is a mother of two and supports her husband Michael in his journey. With a communications degree majoring in journalism, Frankie has worked in media and PR at News Corp and Nova Entertainment, and is now a voiceover artist, voicing many national ads you'll hear on TV and radio. Together Michael and Frankie also own a paint-and-sip studio in the Hunter Valley called Pinot & Picasso.

CONCUSSION

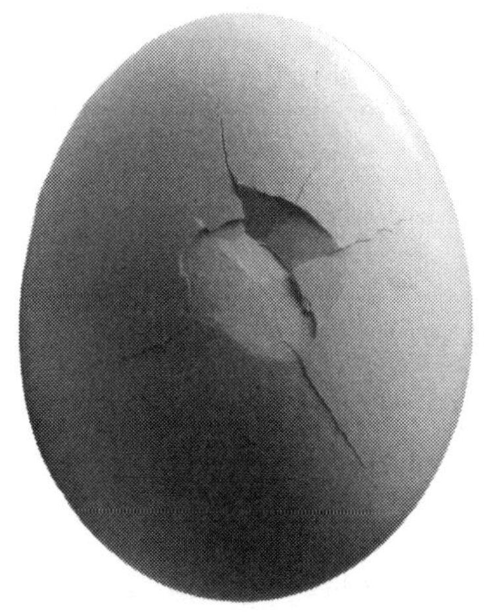

MICHAEL LIPMAN
& FRANKIE LIPMAN

Foreword by Peter FitzSimons

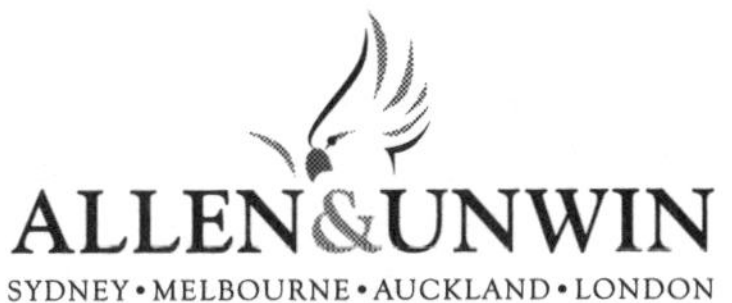

First published in 2022

Copyright © Michael Lipman and Frankie Lipman 2022

All rights reserved. No part of this book may be reproduced or transmitted in any form or by any means, electronic or mechanical, including photocopying, recording or by any information storage and retrieval system, without prior permission in writing from the publisher. The Australian *Copyright Act 1968* (the Act) allows a maximum of one chapter or 10 per cent of this book, whichever is the greater, to be photocopied by any educational institution for its educational purposes provided that the educational institution (or body that administers it) has given a remuneration notice to the Copyright Agency (Australia) under the Act.

Allen & Unwin
Cammeraygal Country
83 Alexander Street
Crows Nest NSW 2065
Australia
Phone: (61 2) 8425 0100
Email: info@allenandunwin.com
Web: www.allenandunwin.com

Allen & Unwin acknowledges the Traditional Owners of the Country on which we live and work. We pay our respects to all Aboriginal and Torres Strait Islander Elders, past and present.

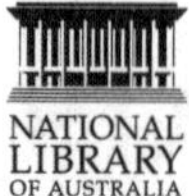

A catalogue record for this book is available from the National Library of Australia

ISBN 978 1 76106 762 4

Set in 12/18 pt Sabon LT Std by Midland Typesetters, Australia
Printed and bound in Australia by Griffin Press

10 9 8 7 6 5 4 3 2 1

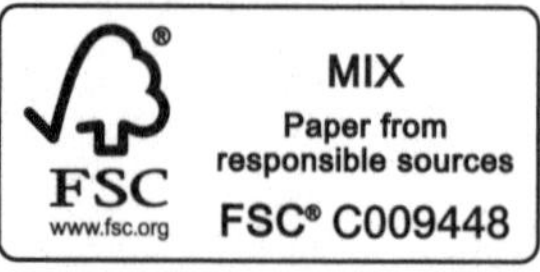

The paper in this book is FSC® certified. FSC® promotes environmentally responsible, socially beneficial and economically viable management of the world's forests.

THIS BOOK IS DEDICATED TO:
Our two beautiful kids, Summer and Joey!
All the families that suffer silently—don't be afraid to put your hand up and ask for help, because there is help and there always will be.

CONTENTS

FOREWORD

Want to, as they say, 'change the narrative'?

We have to see and understand stories that are powerful enough to make key players in the narrative behave differently now and forevermore, leading to an entirely different outcome.

This book contains precisely that: a deeply moving and compelling tale of two people caught up in the consequences of repeated concussions to one of them—a tale so strong that it will help to change the whole nature of contact sports.

And things *must* change.

So far, the narrative on concussion in sport has been a strange one, starting happily and getting incrementally worse as the decades rolled by so that, as we speak, it is no less than an existential threat to entire sports.

In the beginning there was sport, and it was good and it was great, with only the occasional problem emerging through boxers being KO-ed or having their 'bell rung'. They got 'punch drunk'. The rest of us could get badly concussed and only have temporary issues—or so we thought. We could get knocked out on the football field, a bloke would come out with the 'magic water' and a sponge, and we'd be good to go!

Knocked out a week or two later? More magic water. Or, more bizarrely, we'd have smelling salts waved under our nose, in the belief that somehow a quick sniff of something acrid could actually help heal our brains.

I speak for many old footballers now: WHAT WERE WE THINKING?

The answer is, we weren't.

We simply didn't understand that each and every concussion and subconcussion was nothing less than brain damage, and there could be a cumulative effect for some of us that would be devastating. That understanding would come bit by bit as retired footballers and people from other contact sports started struggling, and research revealed this thing called CTE—chronic traumatic encephalopathy—a brain condition found in people who had suffered repeated concussions, leading to consequences such as early-onset dementia.

Did things change immediately in all contact sports because of it?

They did not.

Yes, various 'concussion protocols' were brought in, but while it was one thing to have protocols, it was quite another to have a culture that actually embraced them. More than anything, this book is a close-up account of the damage that can be done by repeated concussions when the protocols are inadequate or non-existent, and the culture is appalling.

I first came across Michael and Frankie Lipman in November 2020, when I agreed to help out Dr Rowena Mobbs of Macquarie University—one of the guiding forces of the National Repetitive Head Trauma Initiative—to research the impact of repeated concussions and subconcussive impacts in sport. My contribution would be to interview a couple of former sportsmen about the effect that multiple concussions had had on their lives since their sporting career had finished.

One of the interviewees proved to be 40-year-old Michael Lipman, a graduate of St Joseph's College and former professional rugby player whose career had included ten Tests for England on the flank as well as a couple of years for the Melbourne Rebels. He came with his wife and business partner, Frankie—*What's doing with her,* I wondered idly as we shook hands, *and why does she look so . . . troubled?*—who is also the mother of their two young children. She had also agreed to be interviewed. In the course of our chat, as the cameras rolled for a video release that Dr Mobbs was making, Michael noted that in the course of his career he was knocked out a staggering more than 30 times, observing that he was part of a culture whereby 'If I wasn't completely knocked out, I played on.'

He was a nice bloke, if slightly withdrawn as he discussed difficult subjects. Like all of us in our early years, he had felt bulletproof—and unstoppable on the rugby field. He had heard of problems with repeated concussions but was sure it wouldn't happen to him. And yet, not long after he stopped playing, both he and Frankie noticed changes in him. He became very forgetful and moody, and he could get very agitated very quickly over trifling matters. Yes, he would quickly apologise, but both she and he sensed that this change in him was not within the parameters of normality.

And it was hard for her.

'Sometimes, you're just walking on eggshells,' she told me with haunted eyes, as everyone in the room leaned in to listen. Consulting medicos, they found their way to Dr Mobbs at Macquarie University, and Michael agreed to be tested. Frankie joined a circle of wives and family members of similarly afflicted sportspeople to give each other support and discuss how to cope.

'There were lots of tears,' she said. 'And once we talked about the effects of concussion, and probable CTE, it was like a light went on. We had all of these answers for everything we had been experiencing.'

And now to the shocking part. Frankie told me that Michael had scored 77 out of 100 in his cognitive tests, which is equivalent to mild dementia.

As you might imagine, I was reeling when I came away from the interview, and I took Dr Mobbs aside in the foyer. 'Doctor, he's forty years old, and getting scores equal to "mild dementia" from concussions in rugby?'

She didn't blink. 'We see many people just like Michael across all sports,' she said. 'This is what we are dealing with.'

And then I contacted Michael and Frankie. 'Great to meet you both,' I said, 'and good on you for having the courage to get help, and being brave enough to speak, but . . . can I write an article about you for the *Sydney Morning Herald*?'

I made it clear that putting the words 'mild dementia' together with '40 years old' and 'playing professional rugby' was going to bring a level of scrutiny for which they had to be prepared.

They discussed it, and Frankie came back to me. 'We are okay with it. That is our situation.'

With their blessing, I put their story in the *Sydney Morning Herald*, and the narrative began to change. A 40-YEAR-OLD footballer has mild dementia from rugby? What is going on?

What is going on is people are now realising that the damage caused by repeated concussions is real and too frequently devastating. And the more people who know about it, the more the narrative can change for the better. Hence this book. My columns have been one thing. But a book that reveals in compelling and horrifying detail the Lipmans' whole experience? It will not only help thousands of other retired sportspeople and their families who are dealing with precisely the same issues, but also give fair warning to current and future sportspeople and their families—get this right, or these are the consequences you face.

You don't need to shut down contact sports. You do need protocols to look after those who do get concussed, and a culture that embraces those protocols to ensure what happened to Michael will happen to few, if any, of those who follow his path. If sports administrators get it completely right, the consequences of repeated head trauma won't happen to any of their players.

FOREWORD

Bravo to Michael and Frankie Lipman for their courage and conviction in recording all of their experiences—the good, the bad and the very, very ugly. I am not sure that we can say it has a happy ending, but at least it has a hopeful one.

Read on. I cannot commend this book highly enough.

Peter FitzSimons AM

1

FRANKIE

First Impressions

2016

Meeting Michael Lipman is not something people forget easily. It's an experience, to say the least. He is the most gregarious, larger-than-life person I have ever known; he blows into your life like a hurricane. Most people thrive off the energy that he radiates, while others misread it and really don't know how to take him. He seems loose, freewheeling, confident, brash and sure of himself, yet also a little . . . unusual. I see it in their faces all the time. I once had a stranger ask me immediately after meeting Michael for the first time: 'Is he bipolar?'

I was really confronted by that question. But at the same time, it made complete sense. Among people you meet in the ordinary course of life, almost no one understands traumatic brain injury (TBI). Hardly anyone is educated about it. We only began to learn what it really means in 2020, when we had to confront the truth about Michael's condition.

Concussion is one thing, but the long-term damage caused by repeated concussions suffered while playing sport—as Michael did for more than twenty years—is a whole new ball game (excuse the pun). TBI is not visible to the naked eye, like a broken limb. Nobody judges you adversely for having your arm in a cast. However, if you suffer from repetitive head trauma and appear uninjured on the outside, you are quickly judged for your sometimes bizarre and erratic behaviour. I know this personally, as I spent many years judging it, without understanding it, myself.

Michael and I met through a mutual friend in a corporate box at a Manly Warringah Sea Eagles rugby-league game in 2016. I will always remember the way he came bounding up to me. One of my closest friends, Emma, once likened Michael to 'an overexcited labrador', and I have never come across a more accurate comparison.

'Michael Lipman!' he announced, offering—somewhat surprisingly but with great assurance and friendliness—a firm handshake. I was the product manager of a News Corp real estate publication, so he pulled out his business card and handed it to me: 'Michael Lipman, Sales Executive, Doyle Spillane Real Estate'.

Instantly I could see how he'd make a good real estate agent. The confidence he had! I was born into the property industry: my dad owned and operated an Elders agency in Collaroy on the Northern Beaches of Sydney for more than 34 years. He had passed away from cancer a little over a year before I met Michael this night and was often on my mind. The fact that my father got his start in sales working alongside Peter Spillane of Doyle Spillane was a huge coincidence. Maybe I took it as a message. I was still grieving deeply and searching desperately for signs that my dad was with me: in rainbows, in songs on the radio—you get the gist. So, I took the synchronicity as a sign that Dad was playing Cupid.

Man, this guy could talk. I'm not sure I got a word in, and I haven't been able to since! I remember at one point Michael said he was 'writing his memoirs', which definitely piqued my interest. Who did he think he was? Ernest Hemingway?

Before long during that first meeting, Michael was doing something a little odd. He had switched to the subject of how the shirt he was wearing was too big for him. He was pulling at it a little frantically and repeatedly asking my opinion. I had known the man for two minutes, and I felt it was a strange conversation to be having, a little 'OCD-ish'. The shirt looked fine to me. He had a great physique, and the shirt fit him like a glove. I couldn't work out what he was going on about. It turns out that he threw it—this perfectly normal and probably expensive button-up chambray shirt—in the bin when he got home that night.

As I was leaving to drive back to my mother's house at Newport, Michael asked if we could catch up sometime. I gave him my number and wondered if I would ever hear from him again. I was a single mother; when I had mentioned this earlier in the evening, he had said that our mutual friend in the box had already told him this and he was pleased to hear it. *We'll see*, I thought. I wasn't holding my breath. The words 'single mum with a daughter' make certain men run for the hills without taking a second glance back over their shoulder.

On the Monday, I was at work chatting with a colleague who was also a good friend. 'Get up to anything on the weekend?' she asked.

I filled her in. To this day, I still don't know who won that Sea Eagles game. I was blindsided by the quirky, charming force of nature who would soon—very soon!—become my husband. I told her about Michael.

'Have you googled him yet?' she asked.

I hadn't. We sat at my desk, and I pulled his business card out of my wallet. 'Hey, I could sell him a page in my magazine' was my rationale for stalking while on the clock for Rupert Murdoch.

I clickety-clacked away at the keyboard, typing in 'Michael Lipman' . . . and with a final tap, I hit the search button. Article after article popped up, and only one or two were related to real estate. Michael had been a rugby-union player with what you might call a colourful past. He'd been an international representative for England, he'd played professionally in England and Australia, and he'd left one of his clubs in controversial circumstances. He hadn't mentioned any of this to me, but suddenly it made sense that he would be writing his 'memoirs'. He'd led an interesting life so far; his history made him seem slightly less of a nut case than the talkative guy I had left plucking at his shirt.

I also found out that he had quit rugby for good, a couple of years earlier, after a succession of bad head knocks. I read about Michael's concussion history before we even had our first date. A year later we were married. I had no idea that chronic traumatic encephalopathy (CTE) was already manifesting itself in Michael's brain, and neither did he.

This is our story.

2

MICHAEL

A Day on the Roller-coaster

2019

I am in my local supermarket, but I don't know how I got here.

It might be afternoon, but when I think about it, it might be morning. Or night. The overhead fluorescents are on, but there are no windows to tell me how light it is outside.

I have a basket of items I must have taken off the shelves, but I can't remember getting them. I feel like I am just waking up from a deep sleep.

In the basket is a packet of tacos, an avocado and a bottle of salsa. I must be making Mexican tonight for the family. I grab hold of the certainty. *Mexican. Tonight.* Okay, I tell myself, what I must be doing now is looking for a tin of black beans.

It's reassuring: I have bought black beans from this supermarket a thousand times. I did it last week. I look to my right and my left. There seem to be a lot of tinned vegetables, but is this the right section? I look up, and the sign confirms that I'm in the tinned vegetables aisle. But should I be in the Mexican aisle? No. If I have the tacos and salsa, I must have been in the Mexican aisle already, and now I've come here for the black beans. Good. Right.

Only, I can't find them. I move carefully past the shelves, my eyes scanning up and down, left to right. Tomatoes, corn, peas . . . beans? There are so many different kinds. I go back to start again at tomatoes, but there are too many different kinds here as well. Chopped, peeled, whole, diced, and so many different brands. I can't handle the tomatoes. I go back to the beans. There are all kinds of beans, and none of them are black.

I know that I've been through this before, and I've got myself out of it. That is one thing I do remember. Sometimes I've gone back and forth, back and forth, again and again, looking for bananas. I spend so much time searching because I'm too embarrassed to ask one of the supermarket staff or another customer. It's humiliating to ask where the bananas are, only to have someone tell you that you've just walked past them for the sixth time.

The dread of going to the supermarket is sometimes so overwhelming that I can't face it. On those occasions I might surprise Frankie by saying—like I've had a sudden inspiration—'Let's have takeaway tonight!' But she knows by now that I'm masking the fact that I'm scared to go to the supermarket in case I find myself in exactly the situation I'm in now.

And it's not like takeaway solves anything. When we're standing at the counter of the restaurant and the person is waiting for our order, I study the menu but can't figure out how to decide what I want. Frankie ends up making my selections for me.

I don't get upset or angry, and I don't burst into tears. Not here, not now. I know how to hold myself in public. I might explode later, or over something else, or when it's the last straw. But not now. At this moment I feel so small with embarrassment, I want to disappear.

'Excuse me, I'm sorry to bother you. I know that there are black beans here, but are you able to tell me where they are?' Time has passed, and I've finally dredged up the courage to ask.

I used to have the courage to run out in front of 80,000 people and a worldwide TV audience, plant my body over the ball, and brace myself for three All Blacks forwards—115 kilograms each—to launch into me like three cars running me over at once. I backed myself to hold my position, take the impact, and secure possession of that ball. If a kick-off was coming to me, I trusted myself to catch that high ball in front of all those people, with those same All Blacks forwards coming full tilt to pulverise me the moment I had it in my hands. I would hang on to it. Courage? It was one of my trademarks.

Now I can't back myself to ask a member of the Coles staff where the black beans are. I've asked a customer.

The customer smiles at me. It's not a generic and polite smile, but one warm with recognition. This is someone I know. I think I can remember her name; I know her quite well, as I see her all the time. She's a parent from my daughter's school. She is, isn't she? No, on second thoughts I might be wrong. She might be someone completely different; she might just have one of those familiar-looking faces. So, I don't say anything.

'Hi Michael, how are you?'

'Hi, ah . . . How are you?'

Something in my sweaty face must tell her that this is not a time for small talk. She must see my desperation.

'Here they are.' She reaches forward, takes a tin out and hands it to me. She says goodbye, and I say goodbye. She was nice enough not to point out that the black beans were right in front of me.

I'm still a young man, and I can't remember what I'm doing in a supermarket. What an idiot.

For five years, I worked as a real estate agent in Sydney. It's not an uncommon occupation for retired footballers. You come out of the game with a lot of contacts and a large network of acquaintances—people who know people—and initially I found it easy to get listings. It wasn't that I was recognised while walking down the street, but within the rugby community I was pretty well known for having played ten matches for England in my twenties. After that, I had come back to Australia, where I had been brought up and started my rugby career. I was a first-grader for the Warringah Rats, and in the last two years of my career I played 22 times for the Melbourne Rebels in the Super Rugby competition before having to retire due to the last of my many concussions on the playing field, this one particularly severe, leaving symptoms that took nine months to subside.

As a start for a real estate agent, a rugby career like that was good enough. Some people liked the reflected glory of dealing with a professional rugby player, and men often loved to hear stories about what it was like to play Test matches on the big stage. I was happy to oblige. I'd gone to a private school—St Joseph's College in Hunters Hill—and prided myself on being able to hold a conversation with anybody, from any walk of life. I was a gregarious person anyway. Pretty much all the attributes for success in real estate.

But in my last couple of years in property, I developed a problem. I would be having a normal conversation with a client about their home, which I was selling, and they'd ask me how the latest inspection had gone. All of a sudden, I wouldn't be able to find the word I was looking for. So, I'd just make up something, clutch at a word randomly. I'd want to say, 'They really liked what you did with the fire pit,' and mid-sentence I'd forget the word for that metal thing in the backyard where you put the wood, light it up and sit around it on a winter's night. So, I'd blurt out something like, 'They really liked what you did with the lighthouse.'

The client would look at me in a funny way. What made it worse was that, in my eyes, I'd be pretending that 'lighthouse' was some sort of private joke that we shared, which gave them an uneasy feeling. Did I say weird things like this to prospective buyers? Could the vendors trust me to act and speak like a normal human being?

Over the last two years of my real estate career, I noticed a steady decline in my listings. In real estate, your income is mostly made up of commissions on the sales you make. You need a certain number of listings to ensure a certain number of sales, and I just didn't seem to be able to develop the same relationships with people that I used to. I couldn't speak naturally. More and more, people were thinking that I was strange, and word got about. What was happening here?

To get me through these increasingly awkward meetings with clients, I started making a lot of notes beforehand, and then carrying the notes in my hand like a script to which I could refer if I lost track. I focused intensely on rehearsing and remembering my lines. Like an actor who had lost his confidence, I just wanted to answer the clients' questions with the correct words, get out of the meeting without having made a blunder, and leave on a good note. Obviously, with this buzzing intensity and the concentration on consulting my notes whenever I was in doubt, my conversational skills were poor. I just couldn't make connections with people anymore.

It reached the stage where I was not getting any new listings, and I couldn't close sales for the old ones I had. I came home and confessed to Frankie that we were about to run out of money. We sold our house in Sydney and decided to move somewhere a lot cheaper: the Central Coast. 'I'll find something to do in manual work,' I said. 'Something where I don't have to remember things.'

I get a job helping out an electrician, Chad. He's the husband of Kirsty, one of Frankie's oldest friends, and he knows that I've struggled since giving up football. He also knows that I took a lot of head knocks and had to stop playing because of them. He knows the history of us moving up to the Central Coast, how I left real estate because I couldn't remember things, and he's sympathetic to our issues.

Chad works with his father, Frank, who taught him everything he knows about being an electrician. On my first day, Frank pulls me aside. 'Electricians get paid more than other trades,' he says, 'because you can die. Whenever you're in doubt about something, just stop and come over and ask us what to do.' Whenever we are on a job together, Chad keeps repeating this message to me. He's a compassionate guy. One day, we're inside a house and he says, 'Hey, Michael, can you go to the van and get me a switch?'

I go outside to his van, open it up and scan the array of equipment in there. It's like the supermarket all over again, except that when I was there I remembered what I needed but just couldn't find it, whereas here I've forgotten what he just told me to get.

Within a few seconds, I'm in a panic. If I don't find this quickly, Chad will think I'm a bloody idiot. He'll come out here and say, 'What's taking you so long?' That's happened before, on other manual jobs I've done since moving up here. Sometimes I've failed at even the most menial work because I can't remember basic things, and I've been too embarrassed to tell my employer or workmate, or they've lost patience with me, or I've lost patience with myself.

Thoughts are flooding my head again, and I still can't remember what I'm looking for.

Eventually, Chad comes out, shakes his head and chuckles, not entirely happy but still understanding. He gets the switch out of the back of the van himself.

But forgetting an instruction can have more serious consequences, as Chad and Frank keep telling me. Another day, when we drive to Newcastle to rewire a whole house top to bottom, I nearly make a fatal mistake.

It's a demanding and stressful job. Chad has to climb under the flooring, into the ceiling cavity, everywhere. He takes me to the kitchen area and says, 'Take the power points off the wall.' He indicates four or five power points. 'Unscrew each one from the wall and leave it hanging with the wires in it. I'll do the rest.'

He provides the instructions in a very clear and straightforward way. But all I process is 'Remove the power points off the wall.'

I unscrew the first two as he wanted and then get distracted by something. On the third one, I remove the power point from the wall, grab a pair of pliers, and then cut the electrical cords.

There is a flare of sparks and a loud zapping noise. I drop the pliers on the floor. Chad runs in. His eyes are popping. Once he's checked that I'm all right, he says, 'Michael, how many times have I told you? If you're unsure about something, ask me!'

'I did what you told me on the first two,' I say.

'So why did you cut the wires on this one?'

I can't give him an answer. My brain just told me to get it off the wall. I lost control, the information was mixed up, and I acted on an impulse.

'You're lucky you didn't die,' Chad says. 'Go outside, go for a walk. I'll take over from here.'

It's a really scary moment. Even with all Chad's warnings, my brain can't process instructions. He could have lost his job. I could have lost my life.

It helps when I prepare people for what to expect. Frankie calls me the king of inappropriate comments. It's just that I have no filter. I've lost the filter I used to have naturally. I do things like asking a friend of Frankie's if she's pregnant, when I know she's not, and I know it's a stupid thing to say. People do that all the time. But I do it *all the time*.

One day we were at my dad's new house, and he was proudly showing it off. I took out my phone and looked up the address on the RP Data website, which collates real estate transactions, and then pointed out some minor discrepancy with the information Dad had given us. It really didn't matter to anyone, except to me in that moment. The king of inappropriate comments strikes again! I'm not one of those people who revels in being blunt, or who enjoys provoking a reaction by disturbing social etiquette. Actually, I hate doing that. But I'm always doing it in spite of myself. What's worse, I don't even know when I'm doing it, and I need Frankie to kick me under the table or make a certain signal to stop me. I didn't do it before, but now I'm the king of it.

When people know me, and know how my troubles are overtaking me, that's obviously better because they make allowances. It's hard for my dad to make allowances for my embarrassing him in front of the family, but at least he knows that this characteristic is new for me. He understands that it's not my real personality, it's something that has come over me in the last few years.

But you can't prepare everybody. In day-to-day life, you're always dealing with strangers who take you as they find you because they don't know your history. Often people don't know how to cope with me when I do strange things. More and more, I need people to show patience with me. But this won't be the case if they don't know me. I don't have a sign on my head saying that I need special treatment, and I don't want one, either. But sometimes I really should have it.

We are at a family pub one day, not long after our move to the Central Coast. It's a comfortable, familiar venue for us; we come here a lot with friends. You can bring children, and it's a nice and relaxed place.

I go up to the bar to order a drink. As it happens, on this day I'm wearing a synthetic-fibre shirt and it's bothering me. It's generating a lot of static electricity, and while it's a loose enough shirt, it's clinging to my body in a way that makes me feel uncomfortable.

A female bartender comes up, and I give her my order. While I'm at it, preoccupied with my shirt, I say, 'I'm sorry you can see my nipples.'

She goes back to pour the drink, and while she's there she says something to another member of the bar staff. I hear this person say, 'Yuck, you've got another guy creeping on you.'

I immediately lose control. Not big time, but I blurt out: 'Did you just say I'm creeping on you? You fucking molls.'

There isn't a big confrontation or anything, but they report me to their manager, who comes over and tells me I'm barred for a year. I'm devastated when I tell Frankie about it. It's going to be detrimental to our social life because we have friends who come here most weeks, and it has a playground where our kids love to spend time. My reaction is not angry but confused. *What the hell did I do that for? It's ridiculous! I never swear at bar staff like that, and 'molls' isn't a word I've ever used in my life! What the hell is going on?*

I think that I have an idea about what's going on. Frankie and I have been dealing with this for all the years we've known each other. We've been dealing with it, even when we haven't known we've been dealing with it.

It's time we know for sure what this is. I need help now.

3

MICHAEL

The Beginning

1980–1998

I have never watched any of the rugby games I played. This is a sport to which I devoted more than twenty years of my life, my best years, my prime. It's not that I don't have access to the vision. Most of the games in my professional career were recorded, and I have DVDs of the Test matches I played for England, as well as some of my appearances for Bristol, Bath and the Melbourne Rebels. It was a solid rugby résumé, by the end. Yet I can't bring myself to sit down and watch any of it. I can't tell you why; there's some roadblock inside my head, and it's not just the fact that I played too many of those big games in a concussed daze. There's something else that's stopping me.

If I want to figure out why, I have to go back to the very beginning.

Although I consider myself Australian, I was born in England. My mother, Janette, had come from a sporting family living on the Northern Beaches of Sydney. Her mother, Margaret, was a talented golfer, and her cousin was Simon Anderson, a world-famous surfer who invented the three-fin thruster surfboard, the configuration used by most surfers around the world to this day. One of Simon's brothers, Mark, swam for Australia at the Olympic Games, and my mother's brother played indoor cricket for Australia. Sport was in the blood.

Mum became a nurse when she left school, and like many young Australians she went to England after graduation to gain experience and see a bit of the world. While she was there, she met my father, Colin Lipman. They fell in love, married and had four children in five years: first David, then me and my twin brother, James, and finally Catherine. Dad was a director in a family business, but they found England a hard place to raise four young children and moved to Australia in 1984, when I was four years old. Dad had been to Australia previously, loved it, and had always hoped to raise his children here.

Australia offered us all a better life. Mum continued with her nursing, and Dad, who remained involved in his family's business, invested in a new enterprise called Painting For Fun. This led to him setting up an art studio and his own business importing and distributing different kinds of paper and other material for artists in Australia. We moved into a typically Australian home on the northern fringe of Sydney. It was located on a steep road called Richmond Avenue in the suburb of St Ives, and my parents had bought the property with the proceeds of the sale of their house in Duton Hill, in Essex, where we'd been living in England. Beyond our back fence and all around us was the Ku-ring-gai Wildflower Garden and the great expanse of what would become the Garigal National Park in 1991.

For us kids, these were idyllic days. We skateboarded on the road or played basketball on the driveway until Mum called us in for dinner. We were all competitive and sporty, willing to give anything a go. I was a high-energy boy, and was asked to chop firewood for the house if my parents wanted to keep me away from more enjoyable activities such as building cubbyhouses, playing backyard cricket and throwing water bombs at passing cars.

We travelled a short distance down Mona Vale Road to go to school at Corpus Christi Catholic Primary School. Between us and the school was Hassall Park, a sports ground where we would go to kick a ball after school. When I got bored, I got up to mischief, once getting caught stealing a couple of magazines from the newsagency across the road from Hassall Park. Always needing to give us something to do, Mum and Dad put us into Little Athletics on Saturdays, which I loved. You got to do everything, from sprints and distance races to discus, hurdling, high jump, the lot. Afterwards there would be a barbecue, and I never wanted to go home at the end of those days.

I can't recall feeling any kind of unease at home, but there must have been tension between Mum and Dad because when I was eight years old Dad moved out. He and Mum eventually got a divorce, and he began living in units in Cammeray, Eastwood and Glebe, before finally settling in Wollstonecraft. Mum had full custody of all four children, and we saw Dad every second weekend. I now wish I'd had more to do with him during my childhood, but it wasn't an amicable separation and we kids were very much a part of Mum's extended family.

Even though we didn't see him very often, Dad's family background had an enormous influence on what happened to me as I grew up.

Until the age of twelve, I had zero interest in rugby. When I wasn't outside playing with my twin brother, or at Little Athletics, I watched a lot of my favourite sport on TV: basketball. This was the 1980s and early 1990s, the heyday of the NBA's influence on kids around the world. Like almost everyone, I was a huge fan of Michael Jordan and the Chicago Bulls, and I would collect cards and fight my siblings for access to the TV when the NBA was on. I played organised basketball and soccer as well as participating in athletics: my brothers were both very good soccer players, while I was tall and gangly but short on skill. James, who was a lot shorter than me, had the fight of a lion in him but could have done with a bit of my size. We didn't play any rugby, and I don't remember watching a single minute of rugby on TV. That was all about to change.

When it came time to send us to high school, my parents decided to pay our way through one of Sydney's top private institutions. They valued education most highly. My brother, David, had started at St Joseph's College (known as Joeys) in Hunters Hill, a boarding school and a virtual academy of rugby. Absolutely everyone played rugby there, and matches involving the First XV were to Saturdays what church was to Sundays.

When James and I reached the end of Year 6, Dad took us to a First XV rugby match between Joeys and St Ignatius' College Riverview. In my head, whichever school won the game was the one we would go to. It was a massive spectacle, with the boys from both schools crammed into grandstands overlooking the rugby field, chanting and singing and making as much noise as they could in support of their heroes. Of course, Joeys thrashed Riverview and that was it for us. Dad actually enrolled us on the basis of the fine school spirit he saw among the Joeys boys, but I created my own memory, which was that it all came down to a rugby result against Riverview. Later, engulfed in school propaganda, we learned to hate Riverview as if it were full of the worst people in the world, little aware that with so much in common—both big Catholic boys' private schools, both members of the elite GPS (Great Public Schools) organisation, both situated on expansive grounds facing each other across the Lane Cove River—the two schools were as close as twin brothers.

The day I walked into the boarding house at Joeys, at the beginning of 1992, was the most daunting of my life to that point. They had separated James and me so that we wouldn't stick together out of shyness, but the result was that in our separate dormitories, neither of us knew a soul.

I was scared as hell. I walked into Dorm B (James was in Dorm A) like a dog with its tail between its legs, already feeling unworthy. I put my bag down next to my bed and introduced myself tentatively to the boy next to me, whose name was David Johnston. I was too shy to say much, but he was the first friend I made. It was a shock: I'd come from a high-energy environment, full of confidence and a feeling of security, to this huge and foreign place. All of my self-belief evaporated just like that.

St Joseph's filled this void with routine and then more routine. Routine governed everything. In the mornings, the lights came on and you had to jump out of bed and line up for the shower with the 40 or 50 other boys in your dorm. You had a minute and a half under the water, and then you were out. If you didn't get in line early enough, this might mean you weren't dressed in time, and then you'd be late for breakfast. In the dining room you lined up and could eat as much as you wanted, but if you didn't finish in time you got a detention. The food was worse than prison grub, disgusting and unhygienic—inedible really—but we were growing boys and had no other option.

Every morning was this almighty rush from one thing to the next. Fall behind, and you got a detention, which meant being held in the dormitory for a couple of hours on a Sunday, the one day we Sydney residents were allowed to go home. It was horrible to have to sit down and write lines when you knew that you could be back playing in the bush or at Hassall Park. Fail a weekday detention, or do something wrong repeatedly, and you weren't allowed out on Sunday at all.

James and I weren't even allowed to be in the same classes. I hoped to see him at breakfast or dinner, but often didn't. This was calculated to make you rely on your friends, your 'brothers for life' as they called them, as a substitute for family bonds. But at first, this meant sitting awkwardly at a table trying to make conversation with the other boys, or just staying silent.

Once classes began, the race to finish on time was intensified still further. There was zero tolerance for a lack of punctuality, so you always found yourself running from class to class, sometimes over long distances, through confusing corridors, and up and down stairs. It didn't matter: it was drilled into you that you just couldn't be late.

St Joseph's was strict on all behaviour. I was frequently sent out of class for not waiting until I was asked to speak to the teacher, or for talking with the other boys. This was the 1990s, but it felt like it could have been decades earlier. The teacher ruled.

The majority of the teachers were Marist Brothers but not actual priests. By then, the only robed priest was the school chaplain. It's hard for me to bring up now, but a couple of the Marist Brothers were very touchy-feely. It certainly was prominent and more or less accepted behaviour. Later, one of them would go to prison. Brother Cyrinus Fisk was notorious for rubbing his private parts against our knees when he was cutting our hair. We said among ourselves that we were going to knee him in his private parts, but nobody ever did. We weren't laughing about it, we were defending ourselves, showing that we were tougher if we stuck together. But if you weren't in a strong group, you were singled out and exposed.

One night in Year 7, I had a nightmare. All of a sudden I woke up, and one of the masters, Brother Ross, was sitting on the end of my bed. It was the middle of the night! What was this bloke doing? He was the Year 7 master in charge, supervising that dormitory, and he had his own room. He'd heard me screaming out during my nightmare, and now he was stroking my leg. I was too scared to say anything because I didn't want to get in trouble, but I also didn't want him touching me. I kicked him and said, 'Go away.' And that was that. But I remember it clearly to this day. He obviously did worse things, as he was sent to gaol. Whenever I thought about it, it raised difficult feelings. I knew what he was doing was wrong, but when you are a terrified twelve-year-old, you also need comfort from adults, and it's possible he wanted me to feel okay.

My positive experiences at St Joseph's far outweighed the small number of negatives. Even though these few unsettling incidents happened to me and others, it was a long time ago now, and I hold the school in such high regard that I would not hesitate to send my own son, Joey, there.

I have to thank the game of rugby for most of my best memories of the school. Survival—and prospering—at Joeys in those days was all about rugby. In hindsight, it seems that the privation and discipline were designed to drive the boys towards a manly group activity where they could protect themselves and feel strong, where they could go outside and let all of their tensions out, and where they could gain status and respect from both their fellow students and the teachers.

There was no TV, and the only sport you watched was school teams playing rugby. As far as I was concerned, rugby was even more of a religion than religion itself.

In my first term, there had been cricket, basketball and tennis on offer, but by autumn there was only one choice. I asked if I could keep playing soccer, but they didn't allow that for under-12s. The rugby coach, a Joeys old boy named Jim Lloyd, asked me what position I wanted to play, and I didn't have a clue. Because I was quite big and fast, he put me at fullback and then in the centres, and he saw something in me that warranted me being in the 12As. To catch up on how to play this unfamiliar game, I stayed behind and practised for hours on end. I'd throw balls against the wall and get the rebounds, practise passing at lunch, try everything I could to get better in what was a competitive environment. You couldn't get me off the training field until I got scared of being late for dinner.

Jim Lloyd saw an energy within me that was unusual. By the time the next winter rolled round, you were allowed to choose soccer, but by now I was fully committed to rugby. According to the mythology of the school, soccer was for effeminate boys who couldn't take heavy physical contact, whereas rugby was for heroes. Seeing that my energy and strength were probably more my forte than passing the ball and evading tacklers, they switched me to the position on the side of the scrum, breakaway (also known as flanker), in the under-13s. I had found my position for life.

Breakaway is the prince of rugby positions: it requires strength, stamina and skill. You have to be everywhere, and very few teams win games if their breakaways haven't played well. As breakaway, you're the fulcrum of the team. You're the driver of the forwards, and you also have to link with the backs. You provide the energy that motors both the attack and the defence. Every other position is highly specialised—the halfback has to be a good passer, the fullback has to catch and kick well, the second rowers must be tall for lineout jumping, and the front row must be built for the low-to-the-ground strength needed in scrummaging—but the breakaway has to be a back and a forward at the same time. The breakaway is the ultimate jack of all trades.

I immediately took to this position. I was in the game all the time. If you're in the outside backs, you do a certain amount of waiting around in rugby; you're not directly involved during long periods of every game. As I had a frenetic personality, I was well suited to the breakaway position where you were always in the thick of the action, limited only by your fitness and desire.

During the under-14s, I started to get serious about my future in rugby. I started to watch the Wallabies and All

Blacks playing each other on TV at home, in the years when the Bledisloe Cup contests were really competitive, and Australia often won the matches. I would sit there studying the players in my position. I studied videotapes of the 1991 St Joseph's First XV highlights. The open-side breakaway, David Kelleher, was one of the best schoolboy rugby players I'd ever seen, and I rewatched the tapes to study his running lines, the way he tackled and how he read the game. I did the same with tapes of Josh Kronfeld playing for the All Blacks, and David Wilson for the Wallabies.

I was also in the basketball Firsts during the summer, but I didn't take it as seriously. I loved swimming and body-boarding at the beach, so I was fairly broad across the chest, but I wasn't a big boy. The thing the rugby coaches and selectors saw was that I had absolutely no fear of any situation or any opponent, no matter what the odds. With the ball, I ran as hard as I could even at the biggest boys. In defence, I took anyone on. The faster or the bigger, the more I enjoyed tackling them. I was just doing what I was doing, not realising I was standing out.

Fearlessness: another word for taking a lot of physical punishment.

My mum ordered me to wear headgear the whole time. I always did. Not every breakaway wore the padded covering, and it wasn't at all what you would call fashionable, but I quickly grew used to it. I think, though, rather than protecting me, the headgear gave me a false sense of my own indestructibility. With the padding, I could lead with my head first. I didn't know then that the only protection it really gave was against superficial cuts and wounds, not the rattling impact on the inside of your skull when you came to a shuddering halt or were whiplashed by being tackled.

I didn't think about that. What I was focused on was playing rugby to the best of my ability. Its high status was constantly reinforced at Joeys by the respect and even adulation it won for you. If you were good at rugby, you were popular in the school. There were all these different groups in the school year, but the rugby guys were the top group. Our team was our own family, and we hung out together. Soon, after such a shy and lonely start in the school, I loved my teammates. I gave them all my heart, and I would have died for those guys. And we were mostly winners. We lost our first game in the 12As against Shore and our last game in the First XV, also against Shore. During the seven years in between, we only lost three games.

When I was sixteen and in Year 11, they elevated me to the Second XV in the open age group. The Second XV was where the First XV coach, Brother Anthony Boyd, put promising players to develop for the next year. It meant I was up against much bigger and older boys, but I thrived on it and made the Firsts when I was in Year 12. I was well respected in the group and took my role very seriously—I was humble, and my focus was all about the team and how we could be the best we could be. We had some good players: Brett Sheehan and Peter Playford were in that team, and they, along with our captain, Alister Campbell, would all become professional rugby footballers. I played against the future Wallaby Phil Waugh in 1997 when he was at Shore, and he was definitely better than me at that age. I'd never heard of him; we didn't pay attention to the other schools, as we were indoctrinated to hate them all.

By Year 12, with so much of my attention on rugby, I'd left my run a little late with my studies. In my earlier years, I'd turned into a bit of a class clown and was given more than my share of Sunday detentions. I didn't get out to see my family much, which was upsetting. I eventually learned my lesson and didn't get in so much trouble, but I was too focused on sport and didn't work hard for my Higher School Certificate (HSC). Rugby and basketball were my world. In 1997, I did the HSC and got something like 46 per cent. I went to Brother Anthony Boyd and said, 'I know I'm not getting into uni with that, so what are your thoughts about my repeating?'

The school was happy to have me for another year, and this time I took my studies very seriously. At the end of 1998, I got 83 per cent in my HSC. The difference was hard work.

For me, the big prize for repeating Year 12 was being made captain of the rugby team. I never captained any team at Joeys until the First XV. One of the other boys said to me, 'We're going to win the GPS comp because we've got you.'

I said, 'I'm not that good.'

He said, 'You have the energy, your work rate is enormous, you're everywhere—you *are* that good.'

It was dawning on me that there was an outside world that I might want to impress, beyond the walls of Joeys. Once

I saw a photograph of myself in the newspaper, which was quite a revelation. It felt like fame. In 1998, we played The King's School at Joeys on the weekend of a huge storm that washed out every other fixture in New South Wales except ours because Joeys had such a fast-drying field among its other superb facilities. The ABC televised that game against the school that was our biggest rival year after year. I wanted to stand out in front of Matt Williams, the NSW coach who was commentating for the ABC alongside Gordon Bray. We thrashed King's, mainly because Peter Playford was so incredible on our wing—he virtually won us that game single-handedly. Kurtley Beale was a freak of nature when he was at Joeys a few years later, but Peter Playford would go close to being the best schoolboy rugby-union player I ever saw. I was privileged to see Matt Burke, Darren Junee, and Tim and David Kelleher in our school colours of cerise and blue, but Peter Playford would have been the best I saw at Joeys.

I knew that I was also a hero to the younger boys in the school. I was that unstoppable guy on the rugby field. Luke Burgess, who would play halfback for Australia, was in Year 7 when I was in Year 12, and he idolised me. He'd come up and ask me how I was. In return, I'd watch him in the under-12s and give him encouragement (the First XV always watched the 12As, and they loved it). The amount of respect we had from the whole school was highly flattering, and if you weren't careful you could get a big head. For that reason, humility was also one of our most prized values.

Being in the First XV, you were already on a pedestal. Being captain was something else again. You had a duty not just to your teammates but also to the whole school to lead by example, to never be in trouble and never be late for anything. You had to do everything perfectly. But it came with privileges: there was some leeway if anything did go amiss. And, instead of eating in the refectory, the First XV would eat at a teacher's house the night before a game, a dinner home-cooked by his wife—always spaghetti—and it was beautiful.

On the Friday night before we were due to play King's in 1998, we were meant to go back to the dorm to study, but I said to the players before dinner, 'In the study break tonight, guys, we're going to meet outside the gates and go to Number One [the field, a kilometre away].' Later that night, we snuck off and sat at the top of the grandstand. I made a little speech about how important this game was, how we'd look back on this for the rest of our lives, and how much it would mean to the school and ourselves. 'Who you are as a person will be determined by those 70 minutes on the field. You've got to reach inside yourselves for something special.' I still remember it. It sends shivers up my spine. It was such a privilege to attend and play for a school like St Joseph's, and the friends I made there are still my best friends. We all see those years as our common touchstone for important and deep feelings of loyalty that remain inside us.

As we snuck back to the dorm that night, we were caught by the Year 12 master, John Reading. 'Everyone else, go inside,' he said. 'Michael Lipman, you stay here.' I waited.

When we were alone, he said, 'Michael, what are you doing? You're not meant to do this.' I waited for the punishment. Instead, he just said, 'Get back to your room!' No way was he going to punish the captain of the First XV the night before a match against King's.

I'd never been a captain of anything before, and now I was making speeches after every game in front of all the parents and staff and players. (We ate as much as we could at those functions because parents would bring platters of food.) In the King's game, I got pulled off at half-time for a corked leg. Brother Anthony Boyd asked me to make the speech at the after-match function, but I was so upset at not finishing the game, I couldn't speak. I was in tears because I hadn't finished. That's how important it was to me.

Important enough to pay a permanent long-term price? The thought never went through my head. Breakaway is a position where you are extremely susceptible to head knocks and concussions. I remember in one game charging full pelt into a ruck to clean someone out, and all of a sudden someone popped up out of nowhere and I got his head or knee or elbow in my face. It was your passion and commitment that made you vulnerable. Your body position was low in attack, your head in the direct path of knees and elbows and shoulders and other heads. Defending, you were doing the same thing but in a different way, with your head over the ball and their heads, shoulders and knees coming at you from all angles, often three at once. Neck trauma and shoulder injuries as well as head injuries go with that position.

But that said, I wasn't often knocked out cold as a schoolboy. Dazed? Dizzied? That would happen most games. Was I damaged? It simply wasn't thought about. As long as I was standing and able to run and had my senses about me, I would keep playing. Nothing would stop me or take me off. Referees and coaches were oblivious to minor head trauma. If you got a knock, they might ask if you were okay, and, of course, you always were. There were plenty of games where I thought, *Gee, I'm not feeling the best, but I can't leave the field because I'll be letting my teammates down.* Letting my mates down was the worst thing I could do. Leaving the field would break the bond; it would be tantamount to saying you didn't value the brotherhood. My loyalty to the team was everything to me. I wouldn't compromise that at any cost.

4

MICHAEL

Taking the Hits

1999–2006

In my nineteenth year, I first came across George Smith. I'd say the New Zealand great Richie McCaw was the best breakaway I ever saw, but the player who had the most talent, who could do everything, was George. I rate him as the best rugby player Australia has ever produced. He could chip and chase, pass behind his back, jump in lineouts, pilfer the ball in rucks and mauls, and tackle anything that moved. He was humble, a lovely man, and he possessed every skill in the book.

George reckoned he only ever got knocked out once in his long career. One hundred and eleven Tests for the Wallabies, 142 matches for the ACT Brumbies, another 201 games for other professional teams . . . and he was only knocked out once. Some people have all the luck.

George and I played together in the NSW and Australian under-19s in 1999, although typically he took the short route into the team while I had a more circuitous journey. At the end of my last school rugby season, when I was the Joeys captain and we shared the GPS premiership with King's and Shore, I was flabbergasted when the Combined GPS selectors picked me on the reserves bench for the Thirds. It was a kick in the guts to be rated the seventh-best breakaway in the GPS competition. Fortunately, the NSW selectors disagreed with GPS, and they picked me out of the obscurity of the GPS Thirds for the NSW under-19s. We won the national championship, I was player of the series, and I was picked in the Australian under-19 team alongside future Wallabies such as David Lyons, Adam Freier and George Smith, and future Super Rugby players Sam Harris and Rudi Vedelago.

We went to Fiji for a game—Mum, who had been born in Fiji, came over to watch—and then played the New Zealand under-19s in a Bledisloe Cup curtain-raiser. The New Zealand team included future greats such as Richie McCaw, Jerry Collins, Joe Rokocoko and Mils Muliaina. I played blind-side flanker while George was open-side. At the end of the game, with us leading narrowly and defending our own line, I managed to hold Jerry Collins up to stop him from scoring. As we were celebrating, George Smith said, 'That's all you, mate.' It was the highlight of my rugby life to that point.

It was also nice to perform well in front of my family, Dad, and his new partner, Lexie, who watched alongside George Smith's family. Riding in the team coach from Stadium

Australia to our hotel would be one of Dad's most cherished memories from my rugby career.

George was my driving force to train harder and be a better player. He'd tell you he was going to the beach, but he'd be lying—he'd be off at the gym. He was an absolute superstar. After we left school, I would butt up against George in the Sydney Colts competition, the under-21 level that precedes the step up to full adult rugby. George had been to Cromer High School and played for the Manly Marlins. I played for their mortal enemies and neighbours, the Warringah Rats. In the year we both played Colts, the biggest game of the year was the beachside local derby, Manly versus Warringah. Early on the Friday evening before that match, my phone rang. It was George.

'What are you doing now?' he asked.

'Nothing,' I said.

He was at my place within ten minutes. George and I had become friends when we played in the NSW and Australian under-19 teams, so we decided to 'test ourselves' by going out drinking that night and seeing how well we could play the next day. (We only did this when playing each other; it was a one-on-one challenge that we didn't replicate with other opponents.)

Our night ended at the Cave nightclub within Sydney's Star City Casino at around 7 a.m. on the Saturday. We were back at my home by 8 a.m., and my mother put us to sleep on two couches, waking us up a few hours later to get us ready to play each other. My mother had moved to her family home in

Woodland Street, Balgowlah, not far from Manly Oval, and George and I walked down the hill on opposite sides of the road with our boots in our hands. Passing motorists tooted us with either encouragement or the opposite.

We walked into our respective changing rooms at Manly Oval and joined our teams for the warm-up and run-on. During the first ruck of the match, George and I were at each other. I pulled on his dreadlocks, he elbowed me in the ribs, and it was on. After the game, which Manly won by a close margin, we got changed back into our going-out clothes and had another night out, this time reflecting on all we'd done wrong.

A year later, George was playing for the senior Australian men's team, the Wallabies, and I was still playing club rugby for Warringah; he really was on another level.

I had joined the Warringah Rats club due to a family connection. My great-uncle, George Anderson, Simon's father, had played for the Rats, so-called because their home ground was built on top of the old Warriewood rubbish tip. I wasn't ever going to play for Manly because I wouldn't get selected ahead of George Smith. And since we'd moved in at Balgowlah, I felt fully part of the extended Anderson family on the Northern Beaches. So, Warringah was the obvious choice.

The Rats were characterised as the battlers compared to the 'silvertails' from Manly, and while those comparisons are often over-egged, there were some extremely hard men at Warringah. Their first-grade forwards, known as the 'Rat Pack', included several club legends, among them Matt Guberina, Rick Black, John Hearn, Dave Purll, Steve Temple and Steve 'Libbo' Lidbury. A number eight who had played for New South Wales and Australia, Libbo was known as an exceptionally abrasive player—which is saying something considering the world of outright thuggery that top-level rugby was in those days. At Rats training, Libbo would turn up for 'Libbo Touch' sessions, games of touch football that became full contact within the first seconds and soon degenerated into open fighting. There was always an altercation when Libbo was involved. We loved and revered him.

There wasn't much violence on the field in my first year at the Rats, when I played Colts, but the next year, when I stepped up to grade rugby, the mentor was another hard man, John Hearn, who taught me how to get away with clever dirty play. Being a big second rower, he was slow around the field, but he made a difference when he got to the breakdown, leading in with his elbows and knees. If there was a hand or an ankle on the ground, he would step on it; it didn't matter who it belonged to, it could be a teammate's or even his own. He had a way of stumbling and accidentally stepping on someone, and he could fall and elbow someone in the face in a way that looked inadvertent to a referee. He taught me how to be street smart. I wasn't a thug, but I looked up to John. He had to bring me out of the clean private-school way of playing I'd learned at Joeys and into the tough real world of men's first-grade rugby. I saw being taught how to hurt people undetected as a blessing. By the time I went to England a year later, it was part of my repertoire.

The nature of rugby in those days meant that outright punching and violence was an inevitable extension of incidental physical contact. Often it was just wild, uncontrolled, blatant violence. There were hardly any send-offs, no yellow cards, no linesmen citing people, no cameras looking at every player from every angle. Taking the field could be more like survival of the fittest. The unspoken motto in Sydney first grade was: 'Get them before they get us.'

I was twenty years old and playing men in their mid-thirties. It was quite an eye-opener to participate in a form of rugby that was more or less amateur, with only two training sessions a week and no video analysis of opponents, yet played with extreme seriousness. Top-level rugby had turned professional half a decade earlier, but the next rung down was pretty rough and ready.

In my two years at Warringah, I was concussed at least once. In a Colts game, I took my headgear off because it had been ripped. Minutes later, *bang!* I suffered a head clash that knocked me sideways. I don't remember much about the concussion, but the wound was spectacular. I had blood all over my face, and the cut later required 25 stitches externally and another fifteen on the inside. The moment was made all the more memorable because my mother and grandmother were watching. My mother was gasping, 'Oh my God, get him off the field!'

Unaware of how horrifying I looked, I was saying, 'Nah, everything's fine.'

My grandmother cut in, hushing my mother. 'What are you talking about? He's fine.'

I went back on the field and finished the match.

While playing for the Rats, I was pouring beers at Manly Warringah Leagues Club, labouring part-time and studying towards a sports science degree at the Australian Catholic University. But I never got beyond my second year at university.

Late on the night of 11 September 2001, a memorable date for many other reasons, I received a call from my agent saying that one of the English professional clubs was asking if I was interested in playing for them. I had previously received an offer from Glasgow, but on my father's advice, I had declined, preferring to wait and see if there was any interest from English clubs.

'Which club?' I asked my agent. He told me it was the Bristol Shoguns, the club of Australian legend Jason Little, Argentina's Agustín Pichot and Felipe Contepomi, as well as a host of fantastic international representatives from the Home Nations including Julian White, Andrew Sheridan and Garath Archer.

I was at the Hunters Hill Hotel, having a drink with my brothers, David and James, and some other mates, watching footage of the unfolding terror in New York City.

I thought about the offer for about two seconds and said, 'Yeah!' I phoned Dad, who agreed that with Jason Little being there, Bristol was a good choice.

I stayed out with my brothers and friends for a big celebration, and the contract was faxed through to the pub; I signed it on the spot and faxed it back. The next day I turned my life upside down, quitting my jobs and my degree.

The invitation didn't come completely out of the blue. It was well known that British and European scouts were trawling through the Australian rugby scene for players who might be eligible, via their parentage, to represent England, Scotland, Wales or Ireland. I'd received an approach from one of these scouts, who had looked into my history and found out that I was eligible for a British passport. I'd discussed this with Mum, who was supportive, as was my father when I told him. My brother, David, was heading off to Europe to work at a Swiss ski resort, and it seemed the time for new horizons.

My flight to England was one of the first to resume after the brief pause following the September 11 terrorist attacks. When I arrived at Heathrow, the airport was very quiet due to the lack of traffic, but there was a news film crew on hand for my arrival—or so I thought. They came up to me with their camera and microphone to ask for some comments. In my complete naivety, I thought they were there for the arrival of Michael Lipman, new recruit to the Bristol rugby club!

In response to their first question, 'How was the flight?', I said, 'The flight was really good. I'm extremely excited to be joining Bristol Rugby and can't wait to start my career there. It's a great opportunity to play with great players. I can't wait to meet them.'

They gave me a funny look and wandered off. I was a 21-year-old airhead with nothing but rugby on my mind, straight out of my cocoon of Joeys and the Northern Beaches. Welcome to the big world. It's not all about you, Michael.

Waiting somewhere behind the news crew, no doubt amused by my gaffe, was a manager and two of the younger players from Bristol. I also met James Grant, a former rugby-union and rugby-league star from Australia who was coming to Bristol as the backs and skills coach. He was going to travel on to Bristol that day with his family, while I piled into a car with the young guys and hurtled along the motorway at 160 kilometres an hour, a speed that had me clutching the door handle.

They moved me into a hotel at first, giving me two weeks to find a place to live. Having been either at boarding school or at home with Mum all my life, I had no idea what to do and was very reliant on the club. In a kind gesture, Jimmy Grant invited me to stay with him and his family until I found a place. I found this to be incredibly generous and we are all still friends to this day. After that, I couch-surfed with some of the players for several weeks before eventually finding a flat in the town.

The 2001–02 season had already started. One of Bristol's flankers, Adam Vander, had suffered a foot injury, and I had been recruited as a backup. Although I was put on the bench for the first few months, playing only Second XV games, the level of professionalism in the club was far higher than at the Rats and I treated every training session like it was a live contest. I fell back on my signature qualities: fearlessness, stamina and nonstop enthusiasm. It didn't matter if my opponent in the training session was a 30-year-old England representative, I tore into him as if it were the last game I would ever play.

Eventually, the First XV coach, Dean Ryan, who I felt had been ignoring me, came up and said, 'I've been watching you. You train like it's a game, and I want to give you a start.'

My debut in a top-grade professional game was at home against Gloucester, and I didn't go very well. At half-time, Jason Little sidled up.

'You need to move faster—you're falling behind the play.'

At first, I didn't understand what he meant. I was as fit as anyone and was racing around the field. I couldn't go any faster! But at this level, rugby is about anticipation and experience, and the best players can see what's going to happen next. You can't keep up if you're chasing where the ball has just been. Jason urged me to think harder about what would happen next, and his advice drove me to pick up my game and concentrate on the flow of play. I turned it up in the second half, and by full-time Jason was more pleased with me. For him to be playing his game and also monitoring where I was showed incredible awareness and rugby intelligence. I certainly couldn't keep up with anyone else's game! But he had played 75 Test matches and won two World Cups with Australia, so I guess he had a head start.

The details of my two seasons at Bristol are hazy now. I played more than twenty times for the Shoguns, and by the end of my second season we were at the bottom of the table and heading for relegation. The owner was trying to sell the club, and there was a lot of flux and unhappiness among the coaching staff as we plummeted from the penthouse in 2002 to the outhouse in 2003.

I recall getting one severe concussion at Bristol. It was a home game against London Irish, or maybe Gloucester. Or was it Wasps? I can't say. During the play, I got knocked out cold—completely senseless. When I came to, I found myself crawling on my knees, trying to chase the direction of play, and then collapsing. I staggered back to my feet, tried to run, and fell over again.

How do I remember this? Only because a few days later, in a team video-review session, the footage of me stumbling about was shown to the entire squad. It was a big joke in the review room. Everyone was laughing about how I was getting up, falling over again, crawling on my knees, getting up, falling over. I guess it was funny, but I wasn't laughing. I was one of the youngest people in that room, and I didn't know what to say or do. The laughter was hard to take, and yet my craziness in wanting to keep playing became a running gag that I felt compelled to live up to. I was that maniac who couldn't be stopped, not even by an obviously serious head knock.

I didn't want to go off the field when it happened, even though it was obvious to everyone that I was cooked. I don't remember any part of the game, not even who our opposition was. But this was rugby, and we were tough men. The frightening and reprehensible thing was that I was allowed to play the following week.

That was the biggest concussion I suffered while I was with Bristol. There were a few others, but none stands out like that one, mostly because of the terrible way it was handled. You couldn't just blame it on the times. Doctors were still doctors, and they had a duty of care then as now. If I was the doctor or coach, even in 2003 I would have said, 'Get him off now.' But instead, I was rewarded for my 'courage' and 'resilience' and given a start the next week.

The reward, I have to add, was huge: big enough to dwarf any thoughts of pulling back and taking more care of my health. From my first season at Bristol, I was already attracting the attention of the England selectors.

It probably started in one of my first games at Bristol, when we travelled to Leicester. They had basically the whole England Test forward pack: Graham Rowntree, Ben Kay, Martin Corry, Martin Johnson and Neil Back were all Leicester players. Not many teams went to Leicester and won. They kicked off. I was 21 years old, and Neil Back might have been 32. In the first ruck, he decided to try to school me. He held me by the face and hit me with his elbow, but he didn't get me cleanly. We began fighting and before long it was me against the entire Leicester pack, which meant the entire *England* pack. It's nothing to brag about. Instinct kicked in, and I was impersonating John Hearn at Rat Park. Because my teammates barely knew me, they didn't really stand up for me. I was left alone in this brawl.

I came off the field racked by disappointment. No matter how a fight starts, it is the duty of teammates to have each other's backs. I lost respect for my teammates. I said, 'You guys always back each other up. That was devastating.' But because I had taken on all of those famous England representatives by myself, I had marked myself out as one of the fearless players. My silly confrontation—and being left in the lurch by my teammates—had ironically marked me out for selectors as a player to watch.

At the end of that season, I was selected to play for an England XV in their traditional fixture against the Barbarians. We were an experimental team of mostly young players, so those hard veterans from Leicester weren't my teammates yet. I was excited by some of the names we were playing against, as the star-studded Barbarians had players from all over the world: All Blacks Jerry Collins and Xavier Rush in the back row, and Springbok World Cup winner Bakkies Botha in the second row. When the two teams lined up in the tunnel for the 3 p.m. kick-off, Jerry Collins was standing beside me. By the look of Jerry, I could tell he (and many others) had had a big night out the night before, which was the custom of the Barbarians during that era. But it didn't faze Jerry, as he had one of the best games I've seen him play—he was everywhere. I loved the game, and it was a highlight of my season, even if the others were not taking it as seriously as they would a Test match. It gave me a taste for more.

While I was back home in Australia after the 2002–03 season, off contract with the now-relegated Bristol, I picked up a deal with Bath. One of the bigger, better-resourced English clubs, Bath had a strong Australian presence in the off-field staff, with ex-Wallabies coach John 'Knuckles' Connolly as head coach supported by Michael Foley, Richard Graham and Brian Smith.

The Bath club had only just avoided relegation the year before, and Connolly was eager to rebuild. This meant that all of the new players had to gel quickly, so there were a lot of barbecues and other social events. I lived with Brian Smith and his wife at first, and let my social side show more than when I was at Bristol. I put on barbecues myself and got to know the other players, who included England internationals Mike Catt, Matt Perry, Iain Balshaw, Mike Tindall, Danny Grewcock, Steve Borthwick and David Flatman, Wales international hooker Jonathan Humphreys, as well as South Africa's Robbie Fleck and New Zealander Isaac Fe'aunati, who acted in the role of Jonah Lomu in the *Invictus* movie. Tim Brasher, the former Balmain and State of Origin rugby-league player in Australia, was also a breath of fresh air when Connolly called him in from running a bar in Calgary, Canada.

Here's an example of the way we handled team bonding. Since a bust-up during a Test match between South Africa and England, Robbie Fleck and Mike Tindall had had a running feud, and there was tension in our squad concerning how the two of them would feel about playing together. The day Robbie arrived in Bath, I suggested we all go out for drinks, as a team, and sort it out once and for all.

Fighting words turned into playful wrestling; soon Fleckie was tackling people in the pub, and we were all kicked out. Fleckie finished the night off by being evicted from his hotel after getting caught running nude through the corridors. He and Mike were fine with each other after those adventures!

Bath is a beautiful city, one of the highlights of England, and the place captured my heart. I loved it there and produced my best rugby for that club. By the end of my first season there, I was selected in the England squad to tour New Zealand and Australia in the middle of 2004. It was a 30-man squad, and the schedule included two Test matches against New Zealand, in Dunedin and Auckland, and then one against Australia in Brisbane. England were the reigning World Champions, and Clive Woodward and Andy Robinson were still running the show as coaches, so it was a daunting set-up to get into.

On the first night of the tour, as decreed by tradition, the youngest player was required to go out with the senior leaders for dinner. At 24, I was the baby, and the elders made sure that a lot of alcohol was drunk. Next morning, when I boarded the team bus, I was hungover and ten minutes late, not a good look. The team captain, Lawrence Dallaglio, sitting at the front of the bus, murmured, 'Eye drops and chewing gum, mate.' They'd initiated me and stitched me up, which was the purpose of the night out.

I confess that I had mixed feelings about representing England, especially on a tour Down Under. I always gave my best to every team I played for, and I had spent three winters in England, but Sydney remained my home. My accent was as Aussie as it gets.

But I didn't realise how confused I was, deep down, until the opening of the Test match against the All Blacks in Dunedin. I was picked on the reserves bench, which meant that, along with the starting fifteen, I lined up on the field for the national anthems. Next to me, Josh Lewsey didn't put his arm around me for the customary team embrace. The anthems were about to start. All he said was, 'You'd better bloody sing this.'

I don't know why, but when the moment came, I didn't sing 'God Save the Queen'. I guess in my heart I was Australian, and my heart was speaking—or refusing to sing—for me.

The high point of that game, and the tour, was what came next. The anthems over, the All Blacks went into their formation for the haka. Carlos Spencer took his position as the leader. Behind him were players I'd either been up against or admired from afar: Tana Umaga, Marty Holah, Keven Mealamu, Carl Hayman and Joe Rokocoko. I thought: *This is it.* It was truly spine-tingling, and I'll never forget that feeling—or I hope I won't. I didn't get on the field that day, but seeing the haka up close was one of the best experiences of my life. *Please God, don't let me forget it.*

As for memories of my first time on the field as an international player, they're already gone. It happened in Auckland, but I don't remember a single detail of it. I remember being presented with my cap at the after-match function, with my twin brother, James, and my mother there for the game, which was special to me, but I recall nothing at all of my England debut. Nor can I recollect much of my second appearance, against Australia in Brisbane, where I had about twenty minutes at the end, replacing Richard Hill. It's all a bit of a blank.

As much as I liked John Connolly, he would leave Bath in 2004. He was replaced as head coach by Michael Foley, the former Queensland and Australian hooker. The next year, Michael's position was taken by the best coach I ever had. Brian Ashton gave us free rein to run the ball from anywhere, even our own in-goal. He hated kicking. 'Why give them the ball back?' he asked. He felt that if the ball was in play you could score from anywhere, so keep it in hand. Quick lineouts, chip and chase, take risks: if they come off, we score. It was a different way of playing rugby, more what you'd think of as Australian than English, which was ironic given that Brian was an Englishman and his liberating tactics went against the Australian John Connolly's much more conservative method. Brian was on his way to being appointed England coach in 2006.

To play that risky style of running, open rugby, there was one painful condition: you had to be super, super fit. John Connolly and Michael Foley had already sent us on Royal Marine Commando training camps for team bonding and to get us to the necessary level of fitness. In training with Brian Ashton, we did a lot of touch rugby and ball skills. Brian accepted that the props could already scrummage, the lineout jumpers could jump, and the halfbacks could pass. 'I'm here to teach you all the other stuff,' he said.

I was blown away. In my element, I produced my best rugby for Brian Ashton. I got my weight down from 104 kilograms to about 100, a big difference when your focus is pace and stamina. The Bath team became one of the great English Premiership sides, everyone performing their role impeccably well, with hardness and accuracy. You didn't have to worry about anyone else not doing his job. We made it clear to each other that if we ever had a chance of winning, we would take chances and go for it. Off the field, motivated to win, we all made sacrifices—no drinking, no distractions, just focusing on being the best players we could be.

My only setbacks under Brian Ashton were injuries, and not just to my head. In February 2005, I injured a tendon in my ankle when the bones separated. I also had plantar fasciitis, some of the worst pain you'll ever go through. I tore the rotator cuff in my right shoulder, which required keyhole surgery and put me out of action for about three months. I was awake during that operation and could see what was happening on the monitor, which was enlightening.

But the head knocks were never far away. During a warm-up game at the start of the 2005–06 season, I was knocked out by an accidental head clash. At the time, I didn't remember what had happened, and I came off because my eye started to close up and I couldn't see. That is, I did not come off because I was concussed. It was a serious enough facial injury that in the ensuing surgery, they had to dislocate my jaw to push my cheekbone back up from the inside and rearrange my face. Because the blood was rushing into my stomach, I projectile vomited all over the nurses when I woke up. I felt so bad that I organised season tickets for them all to come and watch Bath.

With Brian Ashton having been appointed England attack coach, assisting Andy Robinson who had succeeded Clive Woodward as head coach, I knew that I stood a good chance of being picked, having played my best rugby for Brian. I was duly selected for England's 2006 tour of Australia.

The Wallabies beat us comfortably in the first Test in Sydney. I was not on the bench or in the team, and I was also omitted for the second Test in Melbourne. Lewis Moody was a star open-side breakaway for England, and although he had an ankle injury, he was always first choice ahead of me. The 22-man squad for Melbourne was picked on the Wednesday, and for the eight of us who were left out, this meant that our ten-month season was over. We went out for dinner and drinks to 'celebrate' that night, and did the same on the Thursday. On the Friday, we held some pads for the players to charge into during the captain's training run. Then, that afternoon, the eight of us adjourned to Melbourne's Crown Casino.

Around 9 p.m. that night, my mobile phone rang. It was the head coach, Andy Robinson.

'We've had to make a harsh call,' he said. 'Lewis Moody can't play on his ankle. Are you okay to start tomorrow?'

'No problem!' I said. I went back to the roulette table and said to the guys, 'Guess what? I have to go, I'm playing tomorrow.'

'No way,' someone said. Even as I walked off, they thought I was joking.

On the Saturday night, I lined up with my teammates in the tunnel at Docklands Stadium, waiting to run on. The Australians stood beside us, and my eyes darted over to them. Next to me was Mark Gerrard, who had been one of my teammates at the Warringah Rats, and at his shoulder was George Smith.

'Oh no,' George said with a smile.

What I was really nervous about, more than my alcohol intake since the Wednesday, was the national anthems. After Dunedin in 2004, I had received death threats from England fans in the mail and at the Bath club about not singing 'God Save the Queen'. Looking back, even though it was an involuntary action, it seemed childish of me not to force myself to sing. I'd been given an opportunity to represent the country of my birth against the All Blacks. I regret not singing. It was disrespectful. Some people choose not to sing anthems as a statement of some kind, while others sing and burst into tears. For me, not singing was a mixture of immaturity and just having my head so caught up in the coming game that I was too impatient, thinking of my chances of participating at some time in the next 80 minutes, and the moment passed me by.

In Melbourne, I sang 'God Save the Queen' with gusto. That wasn't a problem. The problem was when they struck up the first few bars of 'Advance Australia Fair'. This time, all my effort was concentrated on *not* singing. I tried to block it out of my mind. I'm a very passionate person, and

I was torn. On the inside, I was singing 'Advance Australia Fair' with the 60,000 people in the stadium. On the outside, I kept my lips sealed.

We lost the game, but George and I had our usual great battle. George was one of the top two or three breakaways in the world by then, and his game had gone to a new level since he'd been representing Australia. I came off with about ten minutes to go. I was sober by then: mind over matter! At the post-match function, Mark Gerrard, hearing where I'd been for the previous three nights, said, 'Lippo, you've done it again.' Looking back, I should have prepared more professionally, but having a few drinks when you're not in the 22 and your season is over—you think!—wasn't frowned upon then.

Afterwards, I enjoyed socialising with my Australian mates. Nobody asked why I was playing for England. They knew that I'd gone over to chase an opportunity, and they were pleased for me that it had come off. I felt that there was curiosity from them, definitely not resentment. I would never have been picked in an Australian team ahead of George Smith, and here I was, excited that my international career for England was just beginning.

5

MICHAEL

Something Was Up

2006–2012

Frankie often jokes that I used to 'party with princes'. It's true—once, anyway.

When Mike Tindall and I were playing together at Bath, he was dating Princess Anne's daughter, Zara Phillips, whom he would later marry. He had a birthday party at Gloucester Manor and invited several teammates, along with royals such as Princess Anne, Prince William and his then girlfriend, Kate Middleton, and a young Prince Harry.

Harry was going through his wild period, and over the years I would see him a few more times. He loved rugby and was knowledgeable in conversation about the game. This night at Gloucester Manor, we all had a few drinks and one thing led to another. We got into an equestrian training pit with mechanical broncos, and I ended up putting Harry in a playful headlock.

All of a sudden I felt this iron grip on my shoulder. The royals have permanent security, but you don't know they're there until something like this happens. I turned around, and there was this giant bald security guard saying to me, 'You can't do that, buddy.'

'No problem!' I said. I let Harry go. These were royals, not my mates, and you can't do that.

My confidence was high in those years at Bath. By 2007, after Andy Robinson was replaced as England's head coach by Brian Ashton, I was a regular pick for the national team. I played my first matches in the Six Nations championship at the end of that season. We beat Italy in a stop-start game in Rome, and I was up for a big performance when we went to Paris to play France at Stade de France. I was at my peak healthwise, and my playing form was excellent. We ended up winning, which not many teams were able to do in France. My uncle watched it on TV and said it was just about the best I had ever played. We went down in a tryless game against Scotland in a wet and freezing Edinburgh, and the next week defeated Ireland at Twickenham, a game that Dad thought was my best. I was on a high and feeling confident enough to take a position as one of the team leaders. In a Test against a Pacific Islander team, our guys were a bit timid in contact, maybe even a bit scared of the Islanders. I felt that you had to fight fire with fire, and I led our pack with aggression. We ended up winning.

The following season, in the lead-up to the Six Nations, I was again selected, this time to play the All Blacks at

Twickenham. But the England set-up had changed again, with Martin Johnson replacing Brian Ashton as head coach. My card was probably marked with that change. Martin was a hard personality for me to get close to, and I felt that he had his Leicester favourites—to be fair, the perception was that Brian Ashton also had his Bath favourites, of which I would have been one. If I was good enough, I felt, Martin had to keep picking me. But he was a very different human being from Brian, who made every player feel that they were valued as an individual. Martin was taciturn and generated fear, more of an old-school rugby coach with conservative, old-school playing tactics. There were other flankers around, such as Tom Rees, Lewis Moody, Magnus Lund and Tom Croft, and I knew that I had to be at my very best to hold my England position.

It was exhilarating to anticipate playing New Zealand at Twickenham. Even on English soil, the haka can take your breath away. I was also hyped to be playing against Richie McCaw, probably the greatest open-side flanker in the history of the game.

But early on, something strange happened. In the first ten minutes of the game, I took a hit to the head. Immediately there was a fuzzy horizontal line across my vision, like what you would see on an old malfunctioning TV set. I played for another 40 or 50 minutes with my eyesight impaired. There was no way I was coming off, but I was mentally stressed, more than actually dazed or confused, by this persistent line that wouldn't go away. I didn't play well, and we lost the game. Looking back, it is very scary to think of that weird line across my vision. I should have put my hand up and asked to be taken off, but deep down I knew that if I asked to come off, Martin Johnson would lose respect for me, and I wouldn't play for England again. As it turned out, that's what happened anyway. I was dropped for form reasons, based on that game, and my international career was over.

Not that I knew it at the time, of course. While the event as a whole is a melancholy memory, I also had one of my proudest moments that night. After the game, Richie McCaw came into our changing room on his own. Everyone fell silent. He had his All Blacks jersey in his hand. He crossed the floor, seeking me out, and said, 'I remember you from that under-19s match when you held up Jerry over the line. It stopped us from winning. We hated you, and we haven't forgotten you.'

I later framed his jersey. I was incredibly flattered, and for a little while it masked the disappointment of knowing that I was on the outer with the England selectors.

Still, these patterns only really became clear in retrospect. At the time I was 28 and believed I had five years at the top ahead of me.

I intended to win back my England place with good performances for Bath. I was a very proud club captain by then, a position I shared with Alex Crockett. To lead the team onto our home ground, The Rec, was an amazing honour. The Rec holds 11,000 people and generates phenomenal noise as all of the spectators are close to the playing field. If anything, captaining the team made me play better. We had senior players such as Springboks Butch James and Michael Claassens, and England second rower Danny Grewcock made the job easier. In my first year we also had Jonathan Humphreys, the former captain of Wales, in our team. As captain, I appreciated the senior players more than ever.

We beat Worcester in a Challenge Cup final, which I played a few days after incurring a split lip that required more than twenty stitches. I came off with ten minutes to go because a bit of my flesh was hanging from the stitching. The TV commentators apologised for showing it, as it was truly disgusting. That win was a highlight. After losing many finals, it was great to be able to hoist a trophy. On the flipside, we went to San Sebastian and had an agonising loss to Toulouse in a Heineken Champions Cup semifinal. Walking onto the field, I stopped and looked at the massive, jam-packed arena to take it all in. I turned to the boys and said, 'Let's go.' It was torture how we lost the game. With no time left on the clock, we were holding the lead, and one of our boys took the ball into attack. But it got turned over in the ruck and Toulouse scored in the corner, which they converted from the sideline to win the game. Bliss for the giant crowd but devastating for us!

Injuries dogged me throughout my time at Bath, but until that last year I coped with time off pretty well. Being injured can be mentally and emotionally taxing. You're bored and anxious. You're constantly watching your team, and people are asking you questions about their performances, but you can't help feeling you've been separated from them and are a non-contributor. Once you've recovered and have to win their respect back on the training paddock and the field of play, it's just as challenging. They might love you as a person, but if you've been missing from the game for two months, you're starting from the bottom again.

With this anxiety, some injured players drink a lot, some read a lot, while some visit schools and coach kids, which is what I did. It was my answer to the sheer boredom of the injured player's routine: have coffee, have Nando's, watch a movie, watch TV, go shopping—there's just not enough to do in an English town, even a beautiful one like Bath. I threw myself into the community work to keep moving. When I was injured, I went to schools and functions, making speeches and representing my club. At the Theatre Royal in Bath, I practised with the Tap Dogs so I could perform in a skit for their show. I did a 30-second tap-dancing session on stage. Thank God there's no video of that.

I spent time out at Bath for several physical injuries, but concussion was never one of them. Concussion was treated differently from other injuries: it wasn't taken as seriously because it didn't stop you from running or passing or tackling. Once, when I was concussed and stretchered off in a neck brace, the coach, Steve Meehan, said that all I had was whiplash. He wasn't a doctor. But when I had a head knock, even the actual team doctor would say, 'How do you feel? Are you ready to play? Yes? Then play.'

Most of the time I just rolled the dice. Of course, I was ready to play! I didn't have a broken leg, did I? I didn't want to let my teammates down. I wasn't thinking about the future.

I thought I was all right, but I wasn't. Soon I'd get concussed again. I didn't think about quitting, and the other players didn't discuss the subject. We went to the movies, hung out together and watched games, but we never ever talked about concussion. I never had a consultation with anyone who asked if I had symptoms relating to head injuries. I wasn't the only one. Others were suffering as well. But we all suffered privately.

While I was playing in England, an Australian neurologist named Professor Michael Morgan recommended to my mother that I retire from rugby completely due to my head knocks. He had worked at Royal North Shore Hospital when Mum worked there, and he had treated my brother, David, after he suffered a stroke. Mum contacted Professor Morgan and said, 'My son's had a lot of concussions, and I'm a bit worried about him.'

Professor Morgan replied, 'Michael should retire from all contact sport.' But I had no medical consultation with him—it was just a remark he made to my mum based on his own professional knowledge. In English rugby, where I lived and worked, not one medical person ever recommended that I get a brain scan, much less retire due to the concussions I was getting.

You're a long time retired, and in 2008 and 2009, when the injuries to my body were piling up, all I was thinking was how much I wanted to play for as long as I could. Who wouldn't? I wanted to break back into the England team, and I wanted to win more silverware with Bath. That was the only thing on my mind. I didn't have a degree or a job to fall back on; I didn't know how else to live.

The way my career at Bath ended was painful and controversial. It still infuriates me. I don't care if it tarnishes me, it's that long ago, and I've got no reason not to tell the truth. This story has never been told publicly before.

I've forgotten who we played, but our last game of the 2008–09 season was on a Saturday. We had a debrief in the changing room, and the team went out for a nice night in Bath at the Sub 13 and Blue Rooms bars where we always went.

Then it all kicked off on 'Super Sunday'. We booked a bus at 10 a.m. to take us to London to go to The Church, a popular club—particularly among southern-hemisphere people—that was open on Sunday afternoons. On the bus were 24 of the 30 Bath players, and I would say that more than half of them had taken some cocaine or other illicit substances, though I didn't see them. I had a small amount of cocaine.

We had a great afternoon at The Church, and then all of us got on the team bus to head to the Pitcher & Piano in Fulham, another popular venue where we had a reservation. The Harlequins team was also there, and an altercation took place between Justin Harrison, the Australian second rower who was in our team, and a Harlequins player at around 9 or 10 p.m. Justin ended up with blood all over his face, and I corralled the team together. I got the bus and made sure everyone was on it, and we drove back to Bath.

The next day, we had a Mad Monday in Bath. We went to our clubhouse for a kangaroo court session, a humorous end-of-season tradition in rugby clubs, and then went to a local nightclub. Everyone then said their goodbyes and left Bath for their annual holidays. I was going to Sydney via Cape Town, where I would visit some rugby friends including Robbie Fleck and Bob Skinstad.

The media had got hold of the story about Justin Harrison's fight in London, so there was attention on us for the wrong reasons. It raised eyebrows in the club management, and why wouldn't it? On the Wednesday morning, I got a call from the team manager.

'Michael, can you meet me at the clubhouse at 10 a.m.? I need to discuss the damage that was done here on Monday.'

I didn't know about any damage but went along in good faith. When I arrived, four or five players were there. They told me they'd been called in for the same reason. I said, 'I'm the captain, I can handle it.'

But they insisted that they'd been instructed to stay. The team manager came out and said, 'Okay, you're not here to discuss damage to the clubhouse because there is none. You're here because we want you to take a drug test.'

We were stunned. 'What kind of drug test?' I asked.

'A hair follicle and urine test.'

'We'll give you urine,' I said, 'but it's illegal to take anyone's hair. ASADA doesn't approve that, and they don't even do it at the Olympics.' ASADA was the Australian Sports Anti-Doping Authority; I was guessing that the British equivalent, UK Anti-Doping, followed the same protocols.

The national authority wasn't involved. The Bath club had heard that cocaine was taken on the bus on the Sunday, and they'd commissioned an independent contractor to do these drug tests.

We waited for about an hour, and the drug testers didn't arrive. I said to the manager, 'I'm getting on a flight to Cape Town tomorrow. Let us know when the testers are arriving, and I'll come back in.'

I went home and thought: *This is crazy*. So on an impulse, I hopped on a train and went to a friend's place in London. The team manager kept calling me about coming to the clubhouse in Bath. Ignoring his calls, I was thinking, 'You brought me there under false pretences when you were setting us up to be drug-tested by an independent company in a non-approved way.'

I was aware of their rights and mine. It really pissed me off. I was definitely avoiding the drug test, but the season was over, and I did not believe they were allowed to test for anything other than performance-enhancing drugs anyway.

There was a lot to think about. I'd just signed a lucrative three-year extension with Bath, and I was captain of the club. I had planned to continue doing my best for them, to stay there and coach, and to play more for England. I rang the forwards coach, Mark Bakewell, a guy I really respect. 'Look mate, I'll come back to Bath,' I said, 'but I want a meeting with Bob Calleja.' Bob was the general manager. Steve Meehan, the head coach, had flown out to Australia for a holiday and turned off his phone. 'This has gone all wrong. I've cancelled my flight,' I said. 'I'm coming back.'

On the train on the way back to Bath, I got a call from a lawyer named Richard Mallett.

'Michael, don't have the meeting. I'll represent you. What they're doing is illegal. Don't do the test.'

I said, 'I want to get it cleared and out of the way.' So, I went back to Bath and met with Bob Calleja on the Friday. Two other players were with me. In that meeting was also the players' union representative.

I did the majority of the talking, until Bob slammed his hands on the table and said, 'Michael, I think you should resign.' From this moment, it was clear that the club wanted to get rid of me.

I was flabbergasted when he said that. I stood up, and the two other players and I walked out, leaving Bob and the union representative. Later, I rang Richard Mallett and told him that I was staying put to resolve the situation. The following Monday, I went to a drug-testing company and provided my hair for a follicle sample. The results were negative. I rang Richard and told him about my clean result.

Meanwhile, the players' grapevine was alive with talk about what the club had done to us. We were disillusioned. Could we put our bodies on the line for them again? All the concussions, injuries, blood, sweat and tears . . . after a couple of days of soul-searching, I decided that I couldn't do that for Bath anymore. Richard Mallett put together my letter of resignation.

Soon it was all over the papers. There was so much hostility towards us, I couldn't go out in Bath or do my shopping—I had to get a mate to bring groceries. I was spat on in the street. English fans either love you or they really, really hate you. I used to be a hero in this town, and I couldn't believe how swiftly and savagely they'd turned against me.

The governing body of rugby in England, the Rugby Football Union (RFU), decided to undertake its own investigation. We attended a hearing in front of three members and were represented by our lawyers. We all made statements about what had happened on the Sunday in question. Bob Calleja wasn't at the hearing to give his version, but they called him on the phone. He said that he didn't want me to resign, as I was one of his best players. He was asked where he'd heard the information that players had taken drugs on the Sunday.

A fellow player, someone whom I'd stuck up for over the years, had gone to the club and told them his teammates were taking drugs on the bus to London. He'd told them there was a drug problem in the club, and these players had to go. A 'drug problem'? Four months earlier, another of our prop forwards, England international Matt Stevens, had received a two-year ban for testing positive to cocaine and subsequently quit the club. Maybe that motivated my teammate to say what he did. He then came into the hearing and backed up Bob's version of our meeting: that I had not been sacked, I had resigned without any pressure being placed on me. It was disgraceful.

Two Bath players who did agree to the club's drug test returned inconclusive results and were allowed to continue playing. The RFU dropped all drug charges against me. 'Michael,' the chairman said, 'you're not here because of drugs.'

'So, what's the problem?'

'You refused to take a drug test.'

'But the drug test was illegal.'

'You've brought the game into disrepute.'

I said, 'It's whoever gave them the information that has brought the game into disrepute, not me!'

After all this happened I couldn't look that teammate in the eye, and we never talked again. I thought about the events of the Sunday, and I couldn't remember seeing other people doing drugs. How did he? He'd only picked it up through hearsay, which was how I'd heard about the others, too. People had been too careful to take drugs openly. But hearsay was enough for him to tip the bucket on a large section of his team.

It was handled badly by all parties. Would I have done anything differently? I might have let Bath do the hair-follicle test on me, legal or not, but we were there for hours, and I felt that we'd been brought there under false pretences so I ran out of patience. I got into a bad mood and left. It blew up so quickly, and then it could not be undone.

I went to Cape Town for five days and then flew to Sydney, back to the family home in Balgowlah. The International Rugby Board banned me from all rugby for nine months, for bringing the game into disrepute by refusing a drug test. You see rugby-league players busted for having drugs on them during the season, and they get a one- or two-game ban. Oh well, nothing I could do about that.

So here I was, 29 years old and back living with my mum. In 2010, I went back to my roots and rejoined the Warringah Rats. Rod Macqueen, the former Waratahs and Australia coach, wanted to sign me for the Melbourne Rebels in Super Rugby, but the Australian Rugby Union denied my application. Interestingly, Justin Harrison was playing Super Rugby for the Brumbies. He'd admitted that he'd done cocaine on that Sunday he got into the fight, and he'd copped a nine-month ban as well. Now it was complete, he'd signed with the Brumbies. But my application to play again was being blocked. I couldn't believe it.

Dean Richards, who would become coach of the Newcastle Falcons club, offered me a deal, but I didn't want to go back; I was done with England. I felt embarrassed to walk the streets of any English city.

I was 31 by the time Rod Macqueen eventually got my application approved and signed me on a two-year deal with the Rebels. He was assisted by Paul Ellis, a solicitor and friend of my great-uncle Jonny Anderson. I played Super 15 under Rod, who was a great coach, alongside some fantastic international players, such as Greg Somerville, Stirling Mortlock,

Adam Freier and Mark Gerrard. I loved it. Then, at the beginning of our 2012 season, for our warm-up games we did a tour of England. We played Worcester . . . and then Bath!

So, I was back on my old stomping ground, where (I'd been told) my framed jerseys were still hanging up in bars and restaurants. The day we arrived, I said to Greg, the other senior leader of the Rebels, 'It's a ritual: to get used to the jet lag, let's go out for a team-bonding session and have a good night out.'

We were out until 2 a.m. and I walked back into the Hilton soon after. In the morning, there were cops in the foyer asking for me. I asked, 'What's going on?'

'Apparently you pushed a young man in front of a car and he got hit last night.'

'What the hell!?!' My memory was getting bad by then, but not that bad.

It turned out that this guy had been in a bar where we'd also been, and then he was hit by a car. He wasn't badly hurt. Fortunately for me, it had happened at 5 a.m. I said, 'Great, check the CCTV of when I walked back into the hotel.' It showed me walking in just after 2 a.m.

They said, 'Case closed, sorry Michael.'

Inevitably, the papers heard about it and blew it out of proportion. Lipman's back!

Before that happened, I was going to be captain of the Rebels team for the match against Bath. But because of the attention, I was demoted to the bench.

It was an incredibly nervous day for me. We'd had a good night out, and people had been friendly to me, but I had no idea how I would be received at The Rec. Before the game, I left the changing room after all of the other Melbourne players ran onto the playing field. About 10,000 people were watching. The Rec was like a cauldron.

As I walked out, the entire crowd rose to their feet and started clapping and cheering. They were running down to the fence to shake my hand and have their photo taken. Some of them were so happy to see me again they literally had tears sliding down their cheeks, which made me choke up with pride. The Bath players and coaches came to slap me on the back and shake me by the hand. The game started four minutes late because of all this. My Melbourne teammates were asking me, 'Who are you, what's going on?' Greg and Stirling said they'd never been treated like that when returning to their old clubs, and they'd never seen anything like this before, for any player. They shook my hand, showing their admiration, and I had shivers running down my spine. I felt like the people of Bath had forgiven me. I'd made mistakes, but the punishment was over.

We played the game, and afterwards I went into the public bar of the clubhouse and shouted beers for the hundred or so people there. We had a singalong, and it brought a tear to my eye. From that moment, I could move on. I realised that the majority of people in Bath had felt this warmth for me all along. The reality was so different from what a minority at the club, in the town and in the media had made me believe.

I've been there since with Frankie, and my jersey is still hanging up in various places around the town. I'm respected in that club. Bath is one of the best cities in Europe. I'm so lucky I went back and had my eyes opened to what the people really thought of me. When I'm asked about my rugby career, Bath is the first club that comes to my mind. It was my life, it's in my heart and always will be.

Some people who remember the controversy around my leaving Bath will mix that up with the story of my head trauma. It's not exactly an evidence-based view, as my departure was only about the events of a couple of days. By comparison, over a number of seasons, I suffered repeated concussions and heavy head knocks, as well as countless smaller brain traumas known as subconcussions. Repeated concussions and subconcussions are proven to be linked with early-onset dementia.

Did alcohol play a part in my brain deterioration? The two things often go together because some people self-medicate when they're injured. But my brain impairment wasn't caused by drinking. I never drank enough during my playing days. When I was out with concussions during my time at the Melbourne Rebels, I wasn't going out drinking. I still had to train, do community work and go to games; I still earned my money by fulfilling my obligations to the club. I restricted my alcohol consumption so I wouldn't wipe myself out.

If I'd known of my brain injury, I wouldn't have drunk at all during my career. And I certainly wouldn't have consumed alcohol after I retired due to concussion. I just didn't see the light at that stage. I hadn't come to terms with the fact that I had a permanent injury. I didn't stand back and ask what sort of person I became when I was drinking. It didn't strike me that when I was drinking, I was able to mask what was causing me real pain. You don't want to consider the million thoughts in your head, the irritability, the random comments you blurt out, the mood swings, the confusion. Alcohol makes you feel more relaxed and stops you thinking about the pain you're both suffering and causing. It's common for people with chronic traumatic encephalopathy (CTE) to develop a problem with alcohol, and it often leads to their early death.

My two seasons at the Rebels were a time of healing, and a chance for me to end my rugby career on a bright note. I played 22 Super 15 games for the Rebels. Training in the first season was very hard. We had a rugby-league strength and conditioning coach, who trained us like league players. I was struggling at 31 years of age. You couldn't take a day off training, or you wouldn't be considered for the next game. We trained for hours on end; it was the most brutal training I'd ever done. It went on for a year, not just during preseason.

I don't remember a lot about the games I played for Melbourne. During my last couple of seasons in Bath, I was getting concussed on a regular basis, and at the Rebels I suffered a series of head knocks with major medical consequences. Unluckily for me, I had always been prone to concussions, but by the time I was playing with the Rebels even relatively light blows were leaving me with ongoing headaches, dizziness and disorientation. When I had too many of these major concussions in my second season, and the symptoms didn't recede, I began to fear that if I had another concussion I might not wake up.

It was very hard to retire, and I would have loved to play my last game knowing that I could run out in front of a home crowd and celebrate, as I would have loved to do with Bath. But I didn't get that opportunity. Not many do.

I don't remember getting knocked out while I was at the Rebels. It's a hazy couple of years. I don't remember many games or even my last game. I remember playing the Brumbies early in my first season, but that's about it. Even though my Melbourne appearances are my most recent games, I still don't remember many. My childhood memories of rugby are clear. But I rack my brain and can't remember a bloody thing from about halfway through my time at Bath.

The Test matches, the best days of my life in rugby? Very difficult to recall.

Snippets. Snippets.

By 2012, enough knowledge was out there to treat concussion more seriously. But the main duty of the medical staff at rugby clubs was to check if you could play or not. I had no counselling. There was a doctor at the Rebels who asked, 'How are you feeling today, Michael?'

I replied, 'Same as yesterday. Okay. I got dizzy going for a walk.' I wish that doctor had spent a few hours with me. Her duty of care was done once I told her I wasn't ready to play.

Human anatomy hasn't changed, but concussion only became a big deal once the rugby organisations came under financial pressure from the threat of being sued. The information was out, but they didn't treat it as seriously as they would later. One day they were laughing at players staggering around after being knocked out, and the next they weren't.

It took legal action before they really stopped laughing.

6

MICHAEL

What Now?

2012–2016

After retiring, I had an identity crisis that tore me apart for years. I'd always been known as Michael Lipman the rugby player. Who was I now?

Moving from a professional career into retirement when you're still a very young person is a struggle for most high-level sportspeople, and it certainly was for everyone who I knew when I was playing rugby. And the crisis doesn't stop when you get your first job; it can go on for years. Even now, almost a decade since I played my last game, I am still going through this identity crisis. I look at myself in the mirror and don't know who I am. I know that I'm a loving father and husband who does the best he can. But from my early teens until my early thirties—half of my life so far—I could look in that mirror and see Michael Lipman the rugby player.

All the way through school into adulthood and professional sport, through all the representative under-19s and professional club rugby and international career, I was always that person—not just while I was training or playing, but 24 hours a day, seven days a week. When you excel at something to that degree, particularly if it's in a sport that has a global presence like rugby, you become someone of note. I was never a superstar like George Smith or Stirling Mortlock or Richie McCaw, but I could define myself very clearly by this thing I was able to do better than almost everyone on the planet.

And it wasn't just the way I saw myself—it was constantly reinforced by the way others saw me. When I played at Bristol and Bath, and even (to a lesser degree) in Melbourne, I could walk around the city and people I didn't know would stop me to have a chat about the last game or the next, thc coach, or some other rugby matter. I was asked to do hundreds of appearances at functions, to make speeches at schools or other events, or just to go along and watch. Your mere presence is enough. People want you there to give their event a celebrity gloss. You just ride that wave and don't have to think. Everything is done for you. Your life is engineered by others so that all you need to do is turn up.

Then, in the blink of an eye, it's gone. From one day to the next, you suddenly have to do everything on your own. In my first year out of the game, I was 33 years old and had to learn the basics of living, from doing my laundry and getting a visa to paying my rates. This might sound obvious and elementary to many people, but in my playing days there was a minimum of preparation put into what you were going to do when the dreaded day arrived. You just kicked the can down the road. When I was playing, I can honestly say that I never thought about life after rugby, ever. I'm an optimist. I just thought I'd be okay. That is literally the only thought I had. There was no one saying to me while I was still playing, 'Hey Michael, maybe you should start a uni course, it'll help you later.' I didn't have parents telling me to finish my degree so that I'd have something to fall back on after I came back to Australia from overseas. Everyone was enjoying my success, and a vital part of maintaining that success was to stay in the moment, and not think too far ahead—not think ahead at all! If you wanted to create the perfect plan for heading towards a cliff at the end of your career, you couldn't have done it better than I did.

(Now, fortunately, things have improved. Rugby and educational organisations help players enrol in a university degree that they can extend over a long period, so they obtain their qualification in time for their retirement. Sporting clubs now have work-experience programs that players enter before retirement, which gives them something real to transition into and makes that transition easier. But this was a totally different time. Rugby had only been a professional sport since the mid-1990s, and it went from an amateur pastime—where players did have an outside job—to a full-time commitment in a very short period. It was unprepared, and a generation of players went through a similar shock to mine.)

What makes it even more dismaying for me is that it wasn't as if I couldn't see my retirement coming. In my last year at the Melbourne Rebels, I had a number of cortisone injections for injuries and missed many games due to serious head knocks resulting in concussions. What was I thinking? It was obvious that the writing was on the wall, wasn't it? No: I still wanted to keep playing, and still dreamed of finishing my career on my own terms.

That is what every long-term player hopes for, after all. When I was at Melbourne, Stirling Mortlock got that perfect finish, announcing his retirement and playing his final game before adoring fans and media. Everyone was on their feet in recognition of his contribution to Australian rugby, which had been immense.

In my case, not having a proper farewell was really, really upsetting. I would've loved to have had a fairytale ending at Bath, a club to which I had given the best years of my rugby life. But the Bath story ended with an unpleasant meeting and an announcement to the press before I left in civilian clothes in the dead of night—one of the worst ways to finish your career at a club. When I went to Melbourne, I had hoped to give them my last three or four good years and then go out on my terms. But instead, I spent nine months recovering from concussion before it was agreed—again in an office and not out on the field—that I was finished. To have that farewell moment taken away from you is quite degrading, and unfortunately it left a heavy cloud over my next few years. If I'm honest, I will admit that it still eats away at me.

In 2013, I had a long overdue back operation. There had been a lot of wear and tear to my spine over the previous twenty years, and I had put it off for a long time. Now that I knew that I wasn't playing, I went under the knife, having work done on my lumbar vertebrae and a fusion of my L5 and S1 vertebrae in my pelvis.

In my mind, I thought that the back surgery might just give me a hint of an outside chance of playing again. Rehabbing from it was my sole focus that winter. It was good because it directed my energy to fixing something physical and straightforward. But in a way it was also harmful because it continued my period of denial about what was going on with my head.

And even then, my head wasn't great. I knew that something wasn't right, but I couldn't put my finger on exactly what it was. My perception was foggy, not just in the mornings or evenings but all through the day. My memory was patchy. People thought I was joking around by not being able to remember things the same day they'd happened, and I laughed along, joining the pretence that I was goofing about. I lived my life hoping that everything would clear up by itself.

Then several issues collided. There was the sudden loss of purpose and the waking up to the fact that I did not know what I was doing with my life. There was the equally sudden drop in my physical activity, which went from the extreme levels of a professional athlete (whether playing or rehabbing) to zero, overnight. This had a big impact on me mentally. And then the fogginess and memory blanks were not going away, even though I wasn't getting hit in the head anymore. I went and lived with my mum again, which had its benefits because she is a trained nurse and cared for me very much, but there was also something demoralising in it, as anyone would understand if they moved back in with their parents in their thirties after being independent since the beginning of their twenties.

The game that I love had broken my body and my mind. The crippling back pain didn't stop with retirement and surgery. I had physiotherapy, chiropractic appointments, medication . . . everything you can think of. I couldn't go for runs now. In the mornings I woke up with sore joints. My head was like a scrambled egg. Most of the time I was embarrassed to go out in public, even to the shops or a restaurant. I just stayed at home for a bit, wondering what I was going to do with the rest of my life and how the hell I would find a job. All I'd ever done was labouring, pulling beers at Manly Warringah Leagues Club when I was young, and playing rugby.

It sounds like I was in a mess when I retired, but you wouldn't have guessed that from looking at me. On the surface I was my typical buoyant self.

It wasn't like my generation of rugby players was the very first to go through this. I went out and sought advice from people who had finished rugby. They all said much the same thing: start booking meetings with other ex-players, ask them what they do, build your networks. Just use your contacts and learn what others do. I did that. I caught up with Jason Little, the Wallabies great and former Bristol teammate of mine, who was now the Chief Executive Officer at Goodman Australia, a big company that owns, develops and manages commercial and industrial property. Jason was good enough to take 30 minutes out of his day to have a coffee with me and answer my questions. I met Michael Hercus, another rugby contemporary, who was doing very well in retirement after finishing his top-level playing career in the United States. I met a lot of other ex-players and people they recommended that I see.

I heard people's stories and wondered if I would be any good at what they were doing. But all of these meetings could only take me so far. I could ask someone every question I could think of about what they did, without this process taking me any closer to actually finding a new purpose in life, never mind a paying job. My efforts were genuine, but deep down I was playing a role, following certain steps without having any clear idea where they might lead or what I was doing from day to day.

Realistically, all I wanted was to stay in rugby. At first this meant doing some assistant coaching. I helped Mark Bakewell as defensive coach for Eastern Suburbs, and then worked as forwards coach at the Warringah Rats. But those jobs don't pay a living salary. You do it for the love of the game. I could keep doing it because my money from my professional career was still in the bank, but soon that would run out and I'd need a proper full-time adult job. What would it be?

It came to a head when that money did run out, and I found myself without an income. At that time, I was approached by an acquaintance who was one of the managers at Kerry Logistics, a freight company based at Caringbah, near Cronulla in Sydney's south. I asked, 'What can my role be?' He was a bit vague on that, but nowhere near as much as I was. I hardly knew what logistics were. I 'worked' there for a couple of months but all I did was get taken to functions and meetings as their trophy, the famous ex-rugby player, so they could say they had someone of note working for their company. I had no actual role apart from fulfilling clients' requests to tell them rugby stories at lunches and dinners. The company did try to teach me how to sell the business to potential clients, and how customs clearance worked. But I had absolutely no idea how to give someone a quote on getting a shipping container delivered from China to Sydney, for instance, and I don't think I had any aptitude for that kind of work, either. Eventually, one of the senior people from the company headquarters in Hong Kong flew in and relieved me of my duties. My first thought was: *Thank God.*

Until 2015, I was still drifting. I did a Physical Training course with a view to becoming a professional trainer, but I had no passion for it. I did a bit of labouring, which I saw as something to keep me busy and physically fit between real jobs. Then Tom Baxter, who owned a contracting firm, suggested that I get into real estate. 'You're a good talker, you get along with everyone, and you're always smiling,' he said.

After everything else I'd been giving a go, real estate seemed worth a try. Yorick Sweetnam, owner of Sweetnam's Real Estate on the Northern Beaches of Sydney, took me on for six or seven months before I got a call from Stephen Doyle, a huge rugby fan and the owner of Doyle Spillane Real Estate, another firm near my neighbourhood on the beaches, and he gave me a job. I was able to do some residential sales work with a certificate of registration from a day course I did, but I was short of having a full licence.

For my first two years, I loved real estate. And Tom had been right: meeting people, feeling the thrill of the chase for listings, and making sales formed the sociable, goal-orientated and sometimes high-adrenaline work that I thrived on.

The shadow of retirement was still hanging over me. I would get a boost to my self-esteem from being invited into corporate boxes at big matches to tell rugby stories. But at the same time, I would look down at the field and think: *Jeez, I'd love to strap on the boots, just one more time.*

Just one more time. It's the phrase you hear most often from football players struggling with the reality of retirement. For many of them, if the worst of the post-career injuries they're suffering is a bung shoulder or a dodgy ACL, they can consider it. Many sign up for Golden Oldies rugby with and against players their own age, and they get all the joy of having something to compete for, the thrill of testing themselves and performing at their best for their team, and then the camaraderie of sitting around afterwards and telling each other how brilliant they all were.

I envied even the Golden Oldies because I knew that my history of concussions meant that I would never strap on the boots again. Not even *one more time.* I would have loved that. But the evidence was also clear from my afternoons in corporate boxes or giving speeches at the request of rugby fans. They would ask me to talk about highlights from my career, for England—'What's it like playing the All Blacks at Twickenham?'—or for the Melbourne Rebels or even the Warringah Rats . . . and *I couldn't remember.* I would bluff my way through, speak vaguely, or even make up stuff to cover for the fact that I had no recollection of the things that others remembered so vividly and wanted the inside story about. There was no inside story; there was no story inside me. It was devastating to come to this realisation.

I would see old Warringah players such as David Purll and Steve Lidbury, who had been heroes of mine growing up, and wonder if they were suffering the same memory loss. But I couldn't ask them about it. They were enjoying their status around the club, as I was, too—why ruin it by confessing that I can't remember my games, and asking if they're the same? There's just nothing to gain from these brutal conversations, or so I thought. It's a secret suffering. Men want to pretend they're tough, they won't whinge, and they will do anything to disguise the fact that they can't remember. There are plenty going through it—but we struggle to open up to each other. It's not part of our language.

What I could not talk about with anyone was the accumulation of truly bizarre episodes in which I was increasingly becoming involved. Initially, alcohol played a part, which only enabled me to fob off the incidents as extreme but fundamentally innocuous overreactions to drink.

The stand-out example among several such episodes in those years was the night of my thirty-sixth birthday in January 2016. At the time I was living in a townhouse in Orchard Street, Balgowlah, with my sister and a friend of hers. On my birthday, I went out with a group of mates to the Manly Skiff Club and the Wharf Bar, both on Manly Cove, where we had a few drinks through the late afternoon and into the early evening. I left the Wharf Bar at around 7 p.m.

The next morning, at around 11 a.m., I woke up in my townhouse. My mother was staying over for the night. She looked at me and said, 'You must've been doing pretty well last night, you didn't get home until 5 a.m.'

'I don't think so,' I said. 'I remember getting home much earlier than that.' In fact, I didn't remember a single thing after leaving the Wharf Bar. 'Let me check my phone.'

It turned out that I couldn't find my phone. I thought my sister might have it, so I walked up the street to the cafe where she was working. She didn't have it, but she let me call my number from the phone in the cafe.

A man picked up.

'Who's this?' I asked.

He told me his name and asked if I was the owner of the phone. 'Where do you live?' he asked. 'You can come and pick it up from me.'

We exchanged addresses, and it transpired that he lived three doors down Orchard Street from us. 'I'll be down there in a minute,' I said.

I went to the house and met him at the door. He handed over my phone and gave me a searching look.

'Can you remember anything from last night?' he asked.

'Nothing whatsoever.'

He gave a bit of a sigh as if he wasn't sure whether to take me seriously or not. But I must have looked as genuinely clueless as I was feeling.

'You don't remember, do you?' he replied.

I shook my head. 'Remember what?'

'At four o'clock this morning I found you in the passenger seat of my car,' he said. 'I was up early to go out to do some triathlon training. You were asleep. I went in and said to my wife, "There's a guy sleeping in my car. What do I do? Do I call the police? Do I try to get him out?" I ended up going back to my car and opening the passenger door. You got out nice and quiet, and walked off up the road. I guess you went back home. Later, I found your phone in the car.'

I was too embarrassed to continue the conversation. This must have been when my mum saw me come home. At some point between 7 p.m., when I left the Wharf Bar, and 4 a.m., when this guy found me, I had got almost all the way home and then crashed out in the car of a man I'd never met.

Feeling terrible about the awkward situation I'd put him in, I bought him a nice bottle of Penfolds wine as an apology. Much later, we ended up becoming friends, as we had kids at the same day-care centre. He always found the story very funny to retell, as most people would. At the time we didn't know about my brain condition.

I didn't drink that much before I left the Wharf Bar, but however much it was, it contributed to a sixteen-hour period of memory loss. That's a long time. It was the first time I had an episode of such prolonged amnesia. I laughed it off with everyone else. If it's alcohol, it's funny. If you're suffering the early stages of dementia, it's anything but.

7

FRANKIE

When I Met Michael

2016

I'm not sure how Michael and I didn't cross paths for 35 years. Growing up in Newport, I drove past Rat Park in Warriewood 10,000 times or more. I went to Newport Primary School and then on to Mackellar Girls High School in Manly Vale. Like Michael, I thrived at my high school, and there was never a day I didn't want to hop on the bus and travel the 40 minutes to get there. 'Mackellar Girls Can Do Anything' was our unofficial motto. There aren't too many public all-girl schools in the state, and Mackellar had something for everyone.

Like St Joseph's, Mackellar excelled in sport and produced many Olympic athletes, some of whom came from my era, such as the swimmers Brooke Hanson and Elka Graham, and the world champion surfers Layne Beachley and Pam Burridge (actually, a little before my era!). The school gave girls the confidence to believe they really COULD do anything. We came from diverse ethnic and socioeconomic backgrounds, so there was no elitist attitude at the school. Everyone was on a level playing field. Michael's mother, Janette, was actually in the first enrolment of Mackellar, and we went to the 50-year reunion together in 2018.

I was not sporty at all. I was musical, having played classical piano since the age of four, and was obsessed with the performing arts. If there was a stage, I wanted to be on it. My spare time was spent competing in eisteddfods at the Sydney Opera House, as well as taking dance lessons, musicianship lessons and piano exams. I remember the first year that rugby union was introduced at our school. I did it for one week and played on the wing, until my boyfriend at the time told me to stop playing because he thought I'd hurt myself. I'm 163 centimetres tall, and only weighed 50 kilograms at the time. He was probably right.

I never was exposed to union games (besides my short-lived introduction on the wing in 1997). I was a cheerleader for the Manly Warringah Sea Eagles rugby-league team in 1996 and 1997, so I spent a lot of time at Brookvale Oval, which coincidentally is where I met Michael twenty years later. Fifteen is no doubt a little young to be standing on the sidelines, being wolf-whistled at by drunk men, but my dad was in his element. He was a proud Sea Eagles fan and appreciated the free tickets we received, and I was happy with the $50 we got paid per game! It was all fun and games until a full beer can was thrown at my head during the infamous 1997 Grand Final against Newcastle.

My father took me to my first Sea Eagles game when I was about five or six. I have a vivid memory of the sun being in my eyes as I chanted along with everyone, 'Wally's a wanker,' which was aimed at Wally Lewis. 'What's a wanker?' I remember asking. Dad also took me to every Sydney Kings basketball game with his season passes. We watched the Super Bowl together every year, and were delighted when his home team, the Baltimore Ravens, finally made it—and won—in 2001. Dad loved sport and was exceptionally active himself. He loved cycling and tried his best to get me involved, but it was always a hard 'no' from me, much to his disappointment.

I grew up as an only child, and while I'm sure that this gave me many annoying qualities, it also made me obsess over big families—I always wanted to be adopted into each one I encountered. Dad came from a family of fourteen kids, while in Mum's family there were four kids, and all of my aunts and uncles lived in the United States. So here I was, this only child in Australia, with a huge extended family and no access to them. It's interesting to note that in every one of my relationships, there were four kids or more in each family. I'm not sure whether this was coincidental or not.

My friends used to love coming to my house when we were kids, just to get some peace and quiet. I grew up on Bungan Beach, in a modest 1970s-style beach house; it was split-level, with three bedrooms and exposed beams. The house was probably built to be someone's holiday home, as most houses along the northern part of the peninsula were back then. I had a joyful childhood with my wonderful loving parents, and I spent my days running down the bush track from our front yard to the sand, dodging bull ants and picking freesias to take home and put in a vase. I always had a menagerie of pets. My parents sold the house when they separated in 2007, and my heart ached not only for their relationship breakdown, but also for the only home I ever knew—which was truly magical. It was sold and knocked down by the purchaser from the North Shore, who built a soulless concrete mansion that recently sold again for an area record price. I doubt there are any original homes along Karloo Parade now; it's such a shame.

My father got prostate cancer when I was 23 and lived with the disease for eleven years, until he developed another very rare form called neuroendocrine cancer and died a year after that second diagnosis. It hit him hard and fast. Everyone was so used to him functioning so well with the prostate cancer that no one, including himself, truly believed he would die from the other one. I sat by his hospital bed after some scans came back and the doctor told him that his body was riddled with it and a second lot of chemo wouldn't do anything.

I sat there, fighting back tears so hard I thought I would implode. I couldn't let him see me give up on him. I asked what he needed me to do. 'Just be my cheerleader,' he said.

So, that's what I was until the very end. We never spoke about the inevitable. A few months later, when he was in palliative care, I laid my head on his chest and held him as he took his last breath. My stepmother, my best friend from high school and my stepmother's close friend all stood in a circle around the bed. It was a grief that I had never known before. I was the epitome of 'Daddy's Little Girl'. He was my best mate, and I was his. I was both a daughter and a son to him. My daughter, Summer, was only three when he died, and I am devastated that he never got to meet our little boy, Joey. We named him Joey Stewart Lipman after my father, Stewart Joseph (not after Michael's school!). They say a daughter's first love is her father, and he was truly my superhero, my oracle.

After my father died, my life unravelled. I left my first husband, much to everyone's concern. I was shattered, and I then tore up my own little family. I had my own reasons . . . life is short, as they say. I am not sure my ex has forgiven me and that's okay. I was married to a wonderful man who was, and still is, an amazing father. But the death of my own father left a massive crater in my heart, along with a strong feeling of anger I wasn't prepared for. I wondered what I had done to deserve losing the person I loved so fiercely. My anxiety skyrocketed and I was overwhelmed with a deep sense of resentment. My ex-husband wore all of that pain and I am truly sorry for the way things ended so abruptly.

Dad left me with an absolute administrative mess to fix up with his business. He must have been drowning in guilt and worry before he died, given the situation that he put me and my stepmother in, and I'm sure he was too petrified to speak the truth about certain things that would eventuate once the can of worms was opened. A year and a half later, still with many loose ends not tied up, and bitterness and hurt pulsating through my veins, I was a hot mess. I was not looking for love, I was looking for a distraction. Enter Michael Lipman.

8

FRANKIE

Happy Days

2016–2017

How great is falling in love? I highly recommend it. It's funny what love can make you do. At the start of our relationship, I sat with Michael and watched Hulk Hogan DVDs even though I think wrestling is idiotic and fake. I guess it's like the male version of watching the Kardashians. 'How good is this?' he exclaimed. 'I was obsessed with Hulk as a kid!'

I curled up on his couch in the townhouse he shared with his sister and another roommate, and we watched *WrestleMania III*—to be exact, it was Hulk Hogan versus André the Giant (the 'Best Match of All Time', apparently—body slam and leg drop to seal the win for HH). I honestly believed that Michael proposed to me because of the pain I put myself through in pretending I was enjoying myself. It was like a test.

Another thing I did for love was learn how to play Texas hold 'em poker. I had never played a game of poker in my life, as I thought it was a 'boy' thing, and I loved that Michael wanted to teach me. He taught me well, too, because I learned to smash him. I soon figured out that he was a habitual bluffer, and I could read him like a book. I also learned that he was the biggest card cheat on God's green earth.

I was cautious of introducing Summer to anyone too soon. It was a few months before I felt comfortable that Michael was here to stay. He was really eager to meet her. 'She's a hard nut to crack,' I told him.

'Well, I am the nutcracker,' he replied.

When Summer met Michael, she had just turned five. She was a little Leo, and you would have never met a more competitive five-year-old. We played game after game of UNO, and Michael would never let her win. NOT ONCE. One evening, when she lost her seventh game in a row, she became so infuriated with him that her chubby cheeks grew bright red, she screamed in frustration, and she threw the whole deck of cards in his face. We laughed so hard, which angered her even more, and she stomped up the stairs in a fit of rage, refusing to come down until later on that night.

'Don't get bitter—get better,' Michael would say to Summer. (Now it's our family motto.)

'DON'T CHEAT!' she would scream in reply.

It was the start of a beautiful relationship, albeit a little bumpy at the beginning. However, she can now beat him in cards on her own merit, and all of those hard losses early on have made her wins that extra bit sweeter. I don't have a competitive bone in my body; I end up being a mediator/adjudicator between the pair of them, and I often hear myself saying, 'This will end in tears' whenever we play anything as a family.

We all moved in together in December 2016. Summer was to start school at Manly West Public School the following year. After I had been living in Bondi to be closer to my work in Surry Hills, it was back to the Northern Beaches where I grew up. I was excited to be home again.

Michael had never really had a serious relationship with a woman, let alone with someone who had a child. It was a massive adjustment in his life, and I really should give him credit for how wonderful he was with Summer, allowing for how difficult she was at times. Her reaction was only natural, given that she was a wee little thing who was suddenly living with a man who was not her father. I should have told Michael that of all the nuts, she was a macadamia—almost uncrackable. He tried to buy her love with googly-eyed stuffed toys called Beanie Boos. He brought home at least two per week, until she was drowning in them. She soon learned the art of manipulation and realised that if she got along with Michael, she would be spoiled rotten with toys.

'What's "gotiate"?' she asked us one night at the dinner table.

'Do you mean "negotiate"?' Michael asked.

'Yes.'

'It means to make a deal with someone—to discuss something to get what you want.'

She must have been overhearing his work conversations. I saw her little brain tick over. A lot of 'gotiating' went on between the two of them after that. It was very cute. 'Good "gotiating",' he'd say to her when she would ask for money in return for doing chores, and they would come to an agreed price. Real estate was in her blood, after all.

Michael was desperate to be loved by her. I'd say it took until Joey was born, in 2018, before Summer really committed. Joey was the glue that joined our family together. Summer and Michael now get along like a house on fire. They never argue, and if Summer sees Michael and me squabble, she becomes overly protective of him and unusually affectionate because I think she is so scared of her family breaking up again. They sat together in tears as Michael explained what was happening to his brain. 'I don't want you to change,' she said quietly. My heart dropped to the floor when I overheard them.

Considering that we were married not even a year after we met, and that first period was such a whirlwind of meeting all of his family and friends, I was very lucky that I adored them and vice versa. I loved big families, and it was wonderful to be surrounded by so many people. Michael's older brother, David, and his twin, Jimmy, each have two kids. Jimmy has twins himself! Plus, there were cousins galore, stepbrothers and stepsisters and their kids . . . Summer loved those Lipman gatherings, too. Like me, she loved feeling 'part of something bigger'.

As we got used to those first years together, we did a lot of socialising, lunches with friends, and walks down to Fairlight Beach for early-morning swims before school and work. After a life of driving past Rat Park, I was soon inside watching Warringah play their local derbies against the Manly Marlins. As we lived in Balgowlah, we could easily walk down to the Marlins' oval, and we watched many a rugby game there, too. In the clubhouse afterwards, there were always friendly jibes that Michael Lipman was on Marlins turf. We ate at Hugos on Manly Wharf, watching the ferries come and go, so many times that I can probably recite the menu off by heart. Michael even took Summer and me there before he proposed to us both at a spot overlooking the aquarium and Manly Pavilion, with its gorgeous Art Deco arches on the little headland.

Michael chose this exact spot to propose because one morning when he was going for a run, and in a bad place mentally due to the stress of work, his headaches and the pressure of the new living situation playing havoc on his brain, he stopped in his tracks. The sun's rays had broken though the dark clouds and were shining down onto Manly Harbour, like heaven opening up, and he believes he heard a voice saying, 'Everything will be okay.' Michael burst into tears, openly weeping in front of passers-by. He ran back to tell me that he was sure my dad had just spoken to him. Now, I wouldn't say Michael is what you'd call 'spiritual' or religious by any stretch of the imagination, so I believed that if he said he heard a voice, he heard a voice. It didn't matter that he never met my dad; his certainty about hearing Dad's voice was a clear sign to him that we belonged together.

Fast-forward a few months. He took us to the exact spot, after our Hugos dinner, then dropped to one knee in front of Summer and asked *her* for my hand in marriage.

'Okay,' she said. 'Does this mean we can have triplets now?'

She was desperate for a brother or a sister. Thank goodness that when the time came, only one baby popped out. Two Lipman men in the house was more than enough, thank you very much!

9

FRANKIE

Memory

2016

Given that I met Michael only in 2016, when he was 36 years old and had been retired from rugby for four years, I realise now that he was suffering from symptoms already. Maybe even his behaviour during our first meeting—that strange obsession with the size of his shirt—was itself a collection of symptoms. I honestly thought that the mannerisms were just part of his personality. How was I meant to recognise the symptoms of a disease that neither he nor I knew he had? We didn't even know that the disease existed.

As I got to know him, Michael would often joke, after an example of his unusual behaviour, 'I've had too many hits to the head.' He laughed off his mistakes. Others would also say it about him, in that jokey way, because no one realised what the actual consequences were of having more than 30 major concussions in your life.

'You must be a saint,' I have been told on more than one occasion. 'It's like you have three children.'

'Good luck!' said an ex-fling of Michael's whom we bumped into in Manly one night.

'How do you cope?' strangers have asked.

I fell in love so hard that I ignored it all.

There were times Michael's memory failed, and I mistook these episodes as arrogance or indifference. Sometimes I felt that the things I told him weren't important enough for him to remember, or that my stories weren't worthy of his full attention. He would ask a question, and a common response from me during that first year was, 'I've spoken about this already—you can't remember?' *Maybe,* I thought, *it's just normal male inattention.*

If a friend was telling us something they wanted to keep private, I would say jokingly, 'There's no way Michael will remember what you've been saying ten minutes from now, let alone repeat it to anyone else.' He was like Dory from *Finding Nemo*—he had the proverbial memory of a goldfish. I would watch Michael really struggle with recognising people—not just forgetting names, lots of people do that, but straining to remember people who had been in his life for a long time, such as teachers, former football teammates or clients. I would see the look on people's faces when they had to remind Michael who they were. They were often hurt or annoyed, or, like me at first, they mistook it for a lack of interest. He would forget places we had been just weeks earlier. Conversations, appointments . . . you name it, he forgot it.

Michael proposed to me only a matter of months after we met. It was another example of his impulsive behaviour: he literally woke up in the morning, decided that this was the day, bought a ring and proposed later. It happened so quickly, in fact, that many of my friends thought we were having a shotgun wedding. When we met, I had been separated from my now ex-husband for over a year and a half, but our divorce hadn't been finalised. I was technically still married when Michael popped the question.

This caused all sorts of difficulties, especially considering we had booked the wedding venue and invited guests before I had been granted a divorce. It didn't look like the paperwork was going to come through in time, so we decided to have a commitment ceremony instead—because you can't marry anyone in this country while you're still married to someone else! At the ceremony, our celebrant was going to have to tell our friends and family why ours wasn't a legal wedding. Talk about a bombshell! How the hell do you explain that to everyone?

Michael was furious. 'I can't believe you're still married,' he said. 'Why didn't you tell me?'

I was dumbfounded—we'd had this exact discussion frequently. 'I've told you a thousand times!' I cried in frustration. I felt like I was going crazy; I was starting to second-guess myself. Had we really discussed it all those times, or was I imagining it? Dealing with someone who has an extreme case of bad memory but won't admit to it makes you question your own sanity. There were times I wondered:

If Michael had remembered my marital status, would he still have proposed?

Fast-tracking a divorce is not easy, but it was granted in the nick of time, two days before our wedding. Thank heavens we were able to have a real wedding, not a commitment ceremony.

Our wedding was a big, fun-filled day at North Head Sanctuary in Manly. To add to the excitement, Michael had invited more than ten people whom he had bumped into at pubs or football games or work functions, but he had forgotten to tell me to add them to the RSVP list. We were short-seated and short-plated; people had to squeeze in their bums wherever they could fit. The venue manager had a panic attack when the reception started. Still to this day Michael refuses to watch the full video of his wedding speech; one time he started, but he soon became mortified and turned it off.

In true Michael fashion, he spoke off the cuff. I'm not sure I was even mentioned until the very end when he made all 160-plus guests get off their seats (if they had one) to sing 'You Are My Sunshine', a song my father would sing to me as a little girl. This was a very special detail that Michael *did* remember, and it was a magical moment I'll never forget.

I wish I kept a journal. I love writing and used to keep one when I was young, I'm not sure why I stopped. Luckily, I kept my wedding speech, and even though the act of re-reading it six years later is cringeworthy to me, it brings happy tears to my eyes. Below is what I said after the usual opening of thanking our parents and friends:

> Now, onto the main event—Michael Lipman—my *husband* . . .
>
> You look ten out of ten, as I knew you would. Babe, you are the love of my life. This is what I imagined the 'real deal' to be.
>
> You certainly left an impression the first night we met. Quick shout out to Dave Johnston and Matt Brown—if it weren't for the last-minute invite to the corporate suite at Brookvale Oval, who knows if we would ever have crossed paths? I'm still gobsmacked that it took us 35 years to find each other.
>
> If I ever wanted a sign from my dad that he was up there looking over my love life, well he threw me one as large as the Kings Cross Coke sign. You gave me your business card that night—a real estate agent working in Dee Why. Just like my dad.
>
> The next Monday I googled you at work. As well as a few 'interesting' articles, I found some pictures of your life before I met you, when you were twice as big, had a lot of blood on your face and didn't look one bit like any real estate agent I knew. You left it until the Tuesday to contact me. By this stage I had ruled you out, but then [my friend] Chala got in my head and said, 'Well, he's a real estate agent, maybe you can have some business drinks and see how you go.' Just to clarify, because my

bosses are here, Doyle Spillane has had a longstanding account with News Corp for over 35 years, so when I took Michael as a 'client' to the State of Origin, I wasn't lying—technically!

Back to you, Michael . . . I love, love, love you. You will make the best dad in the world. You already are the best stepdad (officially now) to Summer. There aren't too many people out there who are loved by kids as much as you; you're so much like my dad in this sense. I know that Summer takes pride in you being hers, too. I have loved watching your relationship grow since the first day you met, and you taught her how to flick beer coasters at the RSL. Pretty soon she had crawled into your lap and up onto your shoulders. I feel she has stayed there ever since—it's pretty hard to pry her off you, I must say. You have been so wonderful with her, babe.

As long as you don't teach her how to cheat in card games, I think we'll be okay!

What can I say? You swept me off my feet from the start. I remember in our very early stages you said to me, 'You know we're having kids, right?' I knew at that moment you were 'the one'. Talk about being forward!

I soon learned this is how you are in life. You know what you want, you live life to the fullest and you say what you mean and mean what you say. I have fastened my seatbelt, I know how to put myself in the brace position, and I may need oxygen occasionally (because let's face it, you use a lot of it), but I'm so excited to be on this journey with you.

Speaking of journeys, I will end my speech with a little story about a ferry ride, a phone and a smashed iPad. While these three things don't seem like the usual props for a romantic love story, they will forever remind me of why I love you, Michael Lipman, from the bottom of my heart.

It was a rainy morning. My car had broken down the day before, and Michael was dropping me at the ferry to get to work. We had nearly arrived in Manly when I decided I really needed to take an umbrella. Holding back the expletives, he drove me back home to get an umbrella, to then return me to the wharf.

Out I hopped. Within a minute, I realised I had left my phone in his car. Now, a logically thinking person would have just taken the phone with them, maybe turned it off so as to not get bombarded with calls throughout the day, but not Michael. No, he parked the car in Manly, bolted in his thongs in the rain with phone in hand, pushed past the commuters with no ticket to get on the ferry to hand-deliver me the said phone.

Down the aisles he paced. 'Frankie? Frankie?'

He could not find me—probably because I was still waiting at the wharf, hoping to get my phone back before I hopped on the ferry.

Next thing you know, the ferry takes off. Michael and my phone on it, but not me.

At this stage I had a brainwave and thought I'd ask to use the newsagent's phone to call Michael.

'Babe,' I said, 'you have my phone!'

'Yes, I know,' he says. 'And I'm nearly at Circular Quay . . . Where are you?'

Where was I? I was emailing work from my iPad, which I then dropped and smashed to smithereens on the wet concrete.

Needless to say, we both had faces like thunder when we greeted each other on the other side of town.

Later that day, when he calmed down a bit, he said he thought the whole situation was quite romantic.

Michael, it was your first lesson into my wonderful world of being rushed and disorganised, and still to this day both you and Summer remind me: 'Keys, wallet, phone,' as I walk out the door.

I love that you are crazy and hijack ferries for me. I love that you are larger than life. I love that you are caring, and I see a side of you that some might not get a chance to see. I love how much fun we have together, and I love the fact that I'm standing here right now, as your wife, with the same butterflies in my stomach that were there on date one. Here's to us—may we live each day like our last, and live each night like our first.

Our first dance was to 'Magic' by Coldplay, which Michael chose because he loves a party trick, and cards are his specialty. He only has two tricks, but I must admit they are crackers. Frequently when we meet anyone new at a gathering, he will whip out the cards. And, of course, he will bring them out again even if he has shown you a thousand times already. That's my goldfish.

10

MICHAEL

Alarm Bells

2017–2018

On the surface, things were still ticking along. I met Frankie and fell head over heels. My sister and her friend wanted to move out of the townhouse we shared in Balgowlah. The romance between Frankie and me was still brand new, but I knew that she was the one. I said, 'I love you, so why don't you and Summer move in with me? Let's see how it goes.' So, I went from having no experience in relationships—never having had a serious girlfriend before, let alone shared a house with one—to living with a ready-made family.

Soon we were married, and I had a beautiful stepdaughter as well. We renovated a small three-bedroom townhouse on the Northern Beaches, and before long our son, Joey, came into our lives. I was still connected with the rugby community, which dovetailed well with my job as a real estate agent. I loved going to Warringah games at Rat Park, where I could still maintain the façade of being someone whose life had significance. People who had the hospitality boxes would see me and wave me up; I was somebody again, not just a real estate agent fighting an ongoing battle to win commissions.

But when I look back on those immediate post-retirement years, I see a portrait of a man in denial. If I examined the cause of my issues at all—and I didn't often do that—I thought they stemmed from the grief of not being able to play again, something I was still struggling to digest four years after my final appearance on the rugby field for the Rebels. My motto as a player, ever since I was a teenager, was 'I'm only as good as my next game'. Brother Anthony Boyd drilled that into us at St Joseph's. No matter how well you played last week, it's gone, put it behind you; it's only next week that counts. But in 2012, the next game vanished. And in the ensuing years, the last game vanished as well. No future, no past. I didn't worry about my next game because there would be none. And I didn't worry about my last game because I couldn't remember it.

The first time Frankie began to suspect that something was seriously amiss was on Melbourne Cup Day in 2017.

When we met, times were good in real estate. But there was a slump in 2017 when listings dried up and buyers became hard to close a deal with. A rule of thumb in the residential property industry is that the top 10 per cent of the experienced agents get 90 per cent of the sales commissions. With things contracting, I suddenly found it harder to break in and get new clients than I had in my first two years.

Each day, I was pushing against the current just to try to stay in the same place.

On Melbourne Cup Day that year, Frankie and I went to Hugos restaurant on Manly Wharf with the team from my real estate company. Lunch kicked off around 12.30 p.m., and we had a few drinks, ran an office sweep and watched the race.

For no reason that I could explain either then or now, I went home alone, without Frankie. I am ashamed to say this, but I might have gone into a state in which I completely forgot who I was with and what I was doing. It's just a blank.

When I got home, I greeted Frankie's mother, who was visiting us and looking after Summer. I walked into the kitchen, where she was standing, and said, 'What's going on this morning? What's for breakfast?'

At first she looked at me like she was waiting for the punchline to a joke. Or was I just drunk? But I stood there, steady on my feet, smiling, apparently quite seriously expecting her to answer my question.

She said, 'Michael, it's six o'clock at night.'

I looked outside and saw the sun shining, still quite high in the sky. I was quite rude both to her and to Summer, which was out of character for me, and when I gave Frankie's mum a last look, I didn't pick up how disturbed she was by my bizarre behaviour. I left the kitchen and, overcome by tiredness, went straight to the bedroom, fell on the bed and went to sleep.

I got up sometime later, when I heard Frankie come through the front door. Unbeknown to me, she had been extremely concerned at my disappearance after lunch. She wasn't able to raise me on my phone, so she had wandered from bar to bar in Manly looking for me. Eventually, she had contacted her mother, who had told her I was home and behaving strangely. Frankie picked up some Mexican food for everyone and came straight back.

She was in the process of sharing the food around when I came down from the bedroom. It was like another person had taken control of my actions—and not a nice person. I snatched some nachos out of Frankie's mother's hand and told her that they were mine. I told Summer she was a 'turd'. I was carrying on like a petulant child and was still confused about whether it was morning or evening. I had little recollection of the events of the day. It was completely bizarre, the way I had changed into this other character. Poor Frankie's mother was understandably horrified, and she confided in Frankie how worried she was about my behaviour.

Eventually we got some sleep. And to make that day—the turning point in Frankie's perception of how serious my problems were—all the more memorable, the next morning Frankie discovered she was pregnant with our son.

I do feel sorry for Frankie's mother because she witnessed not one but two of the incidents that woke Frankie up to the possibility that there might be a problem with my brain.

The next one happened a year and a half later, after we had moved to the Central Coast. Frankie's mum was staying with us again. I went for a walk around the block to exercise our dogs and get some fresh air. When I got back to the house, Frankie and her mother were watching TV in the living room.

I began chatting quite candidly with her mum about the walk we'd just taken together. I was continuing a conversation I believed we had been having.

'Michael, I haven't been on a walk with you,' she said. 'I've been here on the couch with Frances the whole time.'

'No,' I insisted. 'We just had a walk around the block together. We had a great chat.'

'Michael, stop joking,' Frankie said. 'She's been here with me.'

I wasn't joking. I could picture every part of the walk, including the presence of Frankie's mother at my side. I sat beside them and stared at the TV, not seeing anything, just trying to piece together the last half hour. I could have sworn my mother-in-law was with me, but I had to take their word for it.

Incidents like this spooked me. I didn't know what was real or what I'd imagined. I still can't understand that frame of mind. Was I hallucinating? I was very disorientated. I'd lost the switch in my memory that distinguishes between what you've done and what you've imagined doing. It was terrifying.

This can't be right, I thought.

My real estate career ended up being broken by what I think of as the stretch between my outer and inner realities.

Outside, I had to be the same smiling, gregarious, fast-talking Michael Lipman that everyone had come to expect of me. Inside, I was literally losing my sense of self.

I treated this with a time-honoured cure: alcohol. I came home from work and got cracking on my evening task: polishing off a couple of bottles of wine. I thought a good drink would make me feel better, but what it did was give me the bravado to do the stupidest thing imaginable, which was to phone clients and try to close deals. We would have a barbecue, I would get on the drink, and my mobile phone would be in my hand. I would call a client and begin gibbering. But I wasn't just a real estate agent getting silly after three or four drinks; I was a real estate agent who kept losing track of words, facts, the identity of the person to whom I was speaking, the address of the house we were talking about . . . in short, anything that could have made such a phone call worth making. I must have sounded like I'd drunk a complete skinful and was mixing it with drugs.

It wasn't just phone calls; it was texts, too. I wasn't making any sense, and, of course, a person who is putting their most prized and valuable asset up for sale is going to be super sensitive to the performance of the agent to whom they've entrusted it. Frankie would watch me working my way through the first bottle and into the second, and she would say, 'Not the best time to message your client.' But she was scared of my reaction because I thought I was fine.

Nobody is fine after drinking that much, and certainly not a person with a history of undiagnosed head trauma. But you couldn't tell me that.

I was spiralling out of control and fighting the pain inside. But clients didn't have to take this into account, and soon they didn't want to deal with me anymore. I always had this voice in my head assuring me that physically I could do anything, I could make sure that everything turns out all right in the end, and I could bring off these sales and save the day at the last minute. But that was not healthy and positive self-talk, it was a kind of hubris to cover the real truth: I was falling apart and failing my family. A deterioration that I had held in check for four or five years since my retirement was now accelerating.

Something had to give.

I started to notice how bad my sleeping was. I would often wake up seven or eight times a night and then lie there for hours, pleading silently for the grace to fall asleep again. I would eventually grow sick of this torture and get out of bed, usually at around 4 a.m. but frequently as early as 3 a.m. I can't tell you the last time I woke up in the morning feeling like I have had a good night's sleep.

I soon noticed the roll-on effect on my mood of poor sleep. It drained the life out of me for the entire day. My energy levels dropped, my mood became irritable, and our family life suffered. I'm known as a fun guy: I would want to go with Frankie and Summer, and then Joey, to the park, or do some enjoyable activity. But if you're only getting four hours of sleep a night on a regular basis, it really has an impact on your mood and your stress levels.

Sleeping tablets were not the answer. I understand that they can work with episodic difficulty in getting to sleep or maintaining a good night's rest, but for me, when the problem became chronic, I knew that temazepam or similar drugs would be bad news: they're addictive and have decreasing effects if you use them regularly. I would take Valium if my back pain was especially severe, but only as a one-off, as this is also a habit-forming drug that may cause unwanted side effects.

Compounding the insomnia was the arrival of crippling headaches in my life. They had started when I was still playing but really intensified around 2014, when I was 34. They came with such disabling pain that I didn't want to leave my bedroom. I just didn't want to go anywhere. My hands would grip my head, I would be in a terrible mood, and I knew that if I left my dark safe room and went outside, sunlight would feel like someone was sticking daggers through my eyeballs. The ache was a persistent pressure in my head that just wouldn't go away, no matter what pain-relieving medication I took. (Forget paracetamol or ibuprofen—they wouldn't even touch the sides.) On days when the headaches were very bad, I could forget about getting a day's work done. Having conversations with people made the headaches much worse. The pressure in my head would become overwhelming, like it really might explode. The pressure was so ferocious that I worried a blood vessel might rupture, or I would have a stroke.

For medical help, I had been going to Brookvale to see my long-term family GP. 'I've got these headaches,' I said, 'and they're definitely due to my rugby career; they only started after I was getting all of these concussions.' The GP referred me to Dr Peter Puhl, a neurologist and neurophysiology specialist, at his rooms in Dee Why. Dr Puhl prescribed the antidepressant Pristiq, starting me on a very low dose, as it could also be used as a pain medication. While he didn't diagnose me with depression, Dr Puhl hoped that the Pristiq would help to eliminate the headaches, as they can be related to stress, anxiety, depression and mood swings. They subsided a little at first but then began creeping up again and intensifying. Dr Puhl increased my dose of Pristiq in response, but we were just managing the problem. It wasn't going away. I had the first of what has turned out to be dozens of MRIs on my brain, to see if anything showed up, but there was no indication of cancer or a stroke or any of the abnormalities that this form of imaging picks up.

I saw Dr Puhl once before I met Frankie and just tried to battle my way along. Things changed dramatically in the two years after we met. Even though I was living with my mother, a nurse, just after I retired from rugby, not much attention was paid to the degeneration of my physical and mental condition in my early thirties. I was focused on getting on my feet after my retirement and achieving something in the transition. Then, after my false starts in employment, my real estate career took off, and I felt that I'd turned a corner career-wise. This led to me denying there was anything wrong. I soldiered on against the headaches, looked for the next opportunity, and if I was in pain and nothing else was working, there was always alcohol.

During our whirlwind start as a couple, my headaches continued the trajectory they'd been on since 2014, growing in frequency and intensity. At first we found another new reason for it: the new living situation. A blended family was a big change for me. Unfortunately, I could be hard to live with. If I had a bad headache and hadn't slept, I was short and irritable and sensitive to the slightest noise. After our first period of the bliss of living together and getting to know each other, it became an incredibly difficult period for Frankie and Summer, and I felt bad for bringing them into this up-and-down life of mine. But still, I didn't think it was a medical problem as such; I just thought I was adapting to life after football and dealing with the ups and ever-increasing downs of real estate. I put my struggles down to the ongoing identity crisis caused by my transition out of rugby. As my property listings fell away, my self-esteem—which is not that high, despite my confident façade—was at rock bottom. I was a constant weight on everyone. Was something really, fundamentally wrong with me?

During that time, I went away for a couple of days. When I came back to Frankie and Summer, I was in the worst mood in the world.

'Have you been taking your Pristiq?' Frankie asked.

'Oh no, I forgot.' It had been three days, and the chemical balance in my brain had switched back to its unmedicated state.

Headaches, mood swings, insomnia and my identity crisis were one thing. Environmental factors such as the stress of my job and dealing with living in a household of three people were another. But forgetting to take my medication was new. Was my memory going?

11

FRANKIE

Walking on Eggshells

2016–2018

After Summer and I moved in with Michael, some days it felt like I was walking on eggshells. Michael would have one of his bad nights and be awake from very early in the morning, and then when Summer and I got up he could not come out of the bedroom, which he insisted on keeping as dark as possible. I would say something, and he would snap at me. I immediately felt that Summer or I must be doing something wrong, and I began to question whether we should have moved in. It wasn't fair on Summer, either. At five years old, how was she supposed to cope with this new father figure who was a bundle of fun one moment, and wouldn't come out of his bedroom the next?

I told Summer that some days Michael was like a big cranky grizzly bear, and we just had to let him hibernate until he came out of it. And he did. During good periods he was the most fun dad and partner, wanting to play with Summer and bubble away with humour and energy. In everything he did, he showed his huge heart and his generous spirit. But then a headache would hit, and a sleepless night, and he would plummet again. I'd ask him, 'Where's the other Michael gone?' He said nothing.

The Pristiq did a lot for his headaches when the dose was right, but then we started to notice the lapses in memory. I'd been aware of Michael's bad memory from the earliest days of our relationship, but I had mistaken it for typical male self-absorption and an unwillingness to listen. He honestly seemed not to remember the information I had given him. Nobody had said to me, or to Michael, that this was the inevitable result of the more than 30 concussions he had suffered while playing rugby.

In 2017 and 2018, I could see Michael's work functionality deteriorate. He'd had some good years in the real estate business, but then he began to come home earlier and earlier. People at his office teased him for knocking off early. It didn't change anything. What was really happening was that he was trying to mask his inability to concentrate. Real estate requires you to make more than 100 phone calls a day. You need to have words at the front of your mind. Michael just couldn't maintain the concentration, and when it lapsed, he covered it up by leaving the office.

He would come home and have a couple of glasses of wine. Suddenly, he felt better! So, he would begin making the rest of his phone calls for the day. Anyone other than Michael could see that this wasn't going to end well.

He left the real estate agency he'd been working for. We thought he was still a gifted salesman—and he was—so he applied for many jobs in the property industry. He would get interviews, but after they saw him, there would be no job offers. It was soul-destroying for him and hard for me, knowing that this charismatic man, a born salesman with a good track record—who just a few years before had been partying with princes in England—was now not even getting a second interview from a real estate agency in the suburbs of Sydney. He was in his late thirties, the prime of life. Yet there was something seriously amiss. He couldn't string a sentence together convincingly when he was under pressure, or he would make up words to fill the gaps.

Michael, being Michael, still persisted with the belief that he was invincible. He just had to pick himself up and go again. Life to him was like a rugby match: you trained, you turned up on time, you followed the processes, you showed resilience when you got knocked down, you threw yourself back into the fray, and you won—or, if you didn't win, you proudly said that you had given it your all. 'I'm fine, leave me alone, there's nothing wrong with me,' he would keep saying, with a shorter and shorter temper, when I asked what had gone wrong with the latest job interview. He batted it off. But I could see something drastic happening, something altogether new. He was losing his impulse control, and even his bodily functions were going haywire. The headaches would go away but then return with a greater intensity than ever before.

Around the time of Joey's birth, Michael was still out of work. When Joey was five months old, I had to go back to my job, which was the last thing we wanted. It was awful watching Michael break, on top of everything else, from the guilt of now being financially dependent on me. I urged him to use his broad network of contacts to find something. 'I know it's not everyone else's responsibility,' I said, 'but you have friends who could get you an entry-level role in the places where they work.' But he couldn't bring himself to ask them. If they had known what he was going through, they might have rallied to help. But he wouldn't open up—how could he open up if he didn't truly understand what the problem was? And so it didn't happen.

'Something's up here, something's wrong,' I said, convincing him to go back to the neurologist, Dr Puhl. He had more MRI scans, which continued to show no sign of cancer or stroke. Medical diagnostics were giving us no answers. And Michael's emotions were getting more and more fragile.

Little things brought him to tears. On one occasion, he was doing some manual work on his best mate's farm up on the Central Coast. But Michael's ability to process information and follow instructions was becoming very limited. While he was there, he was told to clear some scrub, and he accidentally ripped up a valuable olive tree. The friend's wife was really mad at Michael, as the tree was supposed to be a feature. That afternoon, I found him sitting in the lounge room with tears streaming down his face. I said, 'Michael, why are you crying?'

'I've disappointed them so much,' he said.

'We'll just get them a new olive tree, it's not the end of the world,' I said.

But he was inconsolable. He felt that he'd done some terrible injury to his friends. We didn't yet realise that Michael was suffering from a medical condition that was causing his inability to remember and follow simple instructions, as well as his emotional fragility and also causing his self-esteem to crash when he'd done the wrong thing. He was being tortured. And we still didn't know why.

12

FRANKIE

The Turning Point

2018

It was in December 2018 that Michael gave me the biggest clue up until then that something was terribly wrong.

Joey contracted whooping cough when he was only a few months old. I thought that I had been vaccinated for whooping cough during my pregnancy, but it turned out that I hadn't (due to a communication breakdown between me, my doctor and my obstetrician).

We knew that whooping cough could be fatal for infants, so we spent many nights not sleeping. I stayed in Joey's room so I could hear him breathing and monitor his little cough. I would put the tips of my fingers under his nostrils to feel the air going in and out. Fortunately, Joey did not have a serious infection.

When I first heard Joey cough, I mentioned to Michael that it could be whooping cough. He laughed it off. 'Nah—it can't be,' he said, as if he could make it so through the force of his optimism. But I trusted my gut and had Joey tested. When the results came back and showed that Joey had whooping cough, Michael burst into tears. It was the first and last time he would question a mother's intuition.

Joey was recovering from his cough by the time we were due to fly to South Africa for our first overseas family holiday. Having put our home up on Airbnb, we moved into Michael's mother's house for a few days before departing. By then, she was living in a large multilevel home at Avalon Beach in Sydney's Northern Beaches. There was a granny flat downstairs that we bunked into, with Joey in a portacot. Summer spent the weekend with her father, as she did every fortnight.

During this time, a friend of mine had a Christmas dinner for six people at her house at Collaroy Basin. When Michael and I went out together, I was always the designated driver; there was never a question asked. But this day I really wanted to enjoy a few glasses of wine with my friends and relax. Michael, somewhat reluctantly, agreed to be the designated driver. We arrived at my friend's house at around 5 p.m., and after two hours Michael took Joey back to Avalon.

Sometime after midnight, I was still at the dinner. There were only five of us, sitting inside, talking in the living room. Mid-conversation, we looked up to see Michael bouncing in through the door. We laughed at the novelty Christmas singlet he'd put on: an elf.

'Surprise! I'm back!' he announced.

I guess the wine had made me slow to compute what was happening. It took me a minute to register that he was meant to be with our baby, in the granny flat at Avalon.

'What's happened?' I asked. 'Did you wake your mum to tell her you were coming back here?'

Given it was so late, I couldn't imagine him waking his mum. Or if he did, I'm sure she wouldn't have thought it was okay for him to return to the dinner so late and leave her in charge of Joey.

He was silent.

'You didn't tell your mum you were leaving?' I asked. 'You've left Joey alone in the flat, and no one can hear him?'

I started to panic. Sick or healthy, Joey should not have been left alone. Michael just stood there and couldn't comprehend what I was saying. I ordered an Uber and spent the 40-minute drive thinking the worst: that our baby boy was having a coughing fit alone in his travel cot, with no one to hear him struggle. I counted the suburbs left between us and Avalon. Collaroy, Narrabeen and Mona Vale have notoriously long sets of red lights. Once you catch one, you seem to catch them all. It was torture.

We got back to the flat and found Joey sound asleep with his arms beside his head, in one of those zippered suits we would put him in instead of struggling with a swaddle . . . and he was perfectly fine. I felt immense relief, but then it turned to fury. How could I trust this man as a father? How could he be so utterly careless, leaving a sick baby on his own and walking out the door to return to a party? Why couldn't

I have one evening to myself without my husband's behaviour causing me so much worry and forcing me to come home? And yet I STILL didn't understand that Michael was not making these choices deliberately. Instead, his brain was shrinking. His impaired judgement, impulse-control problems, memory loss and confusion were all summed up in this one terrifying episode. But I was still putting it down to his character, not his invisible injury.

I spoke with my friends the next day. Some of them had never met Michael before this night, and they were worried for me. Like me, they had no understanding of what was happening to him, and they thought him reckless and careless. 'Are you sure you've made the right decision being with this guy?' they asked. 'You've got your work cut out for you.'

A few days later, we flew to South Africa. Sometime during the fourteen-hour flight, while Summer and Joey were sleeping, Michael began to cry. 'Summer doesn't respect me,' he said.

'You've got to stop doing such dumb shit,' I said. 'Respect yourself, and she'll start respecting you.'

I knew that he was feeling shame about what had happened a few nights before, but I was still angry because he didn't want to talk about it. And he hadn't apologised. Michael avoided difficult conversations. He was never in the wrong, and if he didn't have to talk about it, then in his head it never happened.

I knew that his tears weren't really about Summer not respecting him. He was aware of the mistakes he was making, and this was starting to take a toll. I agreed to not bring the subject up again while we were away and to just get on with enjoying our holiday. We stayed with Michael's great friends Jules and Johnno, whom he had met while playing rugby in Bath. We also caught up with his ex-teammates during our stay, these wonderful welcoming South Africans we came to consider family. I've never met people like them, so loving, hospitable and caring. And they absolutely adore Michael, as they have ever since he first moved to the United Kingdom to pursue his rugby career.

One night, Johnno pulled me aside and asked if everything was okay with Michael. 'I can see some changes in him,' he said.

It was a conversation I needed to have. I needed someone to acknowledge that something wasn't right, someone who had known Michael longer than I had. Michael's family were not saying anything, but here in South Africa, his old friends noticed immediately. From that time on I could stop beating my head against a brick wall because if others could see changes, then I knew that I wasn't going crazy.

Michael's South African friends were not the only ones who noticed changes. After a weekend at the farm of one of Michael's schoolfriends, the wife had a little chat with me as I was hopping into my car. She knew that Michael and I were struggling and asked if we had considered taking time to go to a mental health clinic.

'I'm not sure I can convince him to do that,' I said, although I knew that the need for help was becoming urgent.

This conversation occurred at a time when we were trying to work out if the cause was alcohol, personality, relationship troubles or who knows what.

'Tell him to think of it as a little holiday for his brain,' she replied. 'Some downtime—although please don't tell him we've had this conversation.'

A little holiday for his brain. When the time came for Michael to eventually speak out and say he needed some serious help, and he was worried what people would think of him going to a mental health clinic, I repeated this line. 'Firstly, no one has to know you are going,' I said. 'And secondly, think of it as a little holiday for your brain. I would go if I could or needed to.'

His thinking began to shift.

13

MICHAEL

Facing the Unknown

2019

By 2019, we were running out of money. Sydney is an expensive place to live, and like a lot of people we found ourselves in a situation where we were asset-rich but cash-poor. We owned our townhouse in Balgowlah but didn't have enough money coming in to pay our expenses. So, we sold the townhouse and bought a cheaper place on the Central Coast, two hours north of Sydney. It was the only way to free up some funds until things turned around for me.

After the decline of my real estate career and my continuing inability to get a new job, we realised that maybe office work wasn't for me. I'd been out of work for four or five months, and I thought that a change of location might trigger a change in the way I was thinking about my working life. Frankie was doing PR for a property developer, and through them she got me a job as a labourer on building sites. They saw that I was strong and fit, had a good work ethic and got on well with people. It was nice working in the fresh air, and I wouldn't have to deal with computers or documentation or all of the communication issues I had struggled with while working in a real estate office. To become a manual labourer at the age of 39 was a kick in the guts, but we were out of Sydney and nobody knew who I was, so the drop in status wasn't rubbed in my face. At first, moving to the Central Coast and becoming a labourer gave me a new lease on life.

Also, around that time, I started a new medication. Desvenlafaxine is the active ingredient in Pristiq, but in a new form it changed my life. For a start, it got me out of the bedroom every morning. I could go running, I could use my body to work, I could leave the house and lead a normal life. I was a totally different person. I'd been really struggling physically, and the right medication laid a foundation for me to get my body moving and rebuild my self-respect by going out and earning a wage.

I was now taking a long list of medications, however, and that fact was not making me happy. It felt terrible to know that I was dependent on these drugs. I needed Endone, a strong painkiller, to numb the physical pain in my back so I could get through a day's work. Becoming dependent on painkilling drugs was a constant worry, but if that was what it took to get me to work, then I would choose to take the pills. I needed to feel like I had earned something that day, done something between sunrise and sunset to make that day worth living. By the end of it, I could look at myself in the mirror and say,

'You're okay mate; you're not dead. You didn't sit around watching TV or doing nothing today. You looked after your family.'

Ultimately, however, this was just a physical thing. I could get my body working again. But even with manual work, you need to be able to think. I found myself constantly making mistakes because I was unable to remember and follow instructions. I learned to put aside my bravado and always say to people before I started something, 'Please be very specific, even over-specific, in the instructions you give me. Otherwise, I'll mess up and walk out.' But even when I was given specific instructions, I would still sometimes forget them, and then I would be too ashamed to ask the person to repeat what they'd told me just a few minutes before. Covering up my humiliation only led to more mistakes. The incident with my friends' olive tree was just one of many. And when each stuff-up occurred, it wouldn't take me long to catastrophise it.

'You've done it again,' I would tell myself. 'You stuff up everything you touch.'

Every time I made a small mistake at work, it felt like the end of the world. *You're a loser.* Little things brought me down like I had a tonne of bricks on top of me and I couldn't escape. I tried to complete an online building and construction diploma, but I stopped the course midway through when I just couldn't force my brain to concentrate. *You're a non-achiever, a failure, you can't even function properly as a builder's labourer. You used to be the guy everyone wanted to be with, the light in their lives. Now you're a burden on everyone.* I think deep down I'm a decent and nice person, but I hurt the people I loved most on a daily basis, which was the hardest thing.

And then I started losing my spatial awareness.

One early sign of this was a pair of car accidents I caused, three months apart, not long after we had moved to the Central Coast. Coming home in the car, in daylight hours, I drove into the telegraph pole beside our driveway. There was no explanation other than my mind was elsewhere. I can't describe it as anything other than a temporary loss of awareness. It's bizarre, just driving into a telegraph pole for no reason at all. I was so ashamed of myself that I didn't tell Frankie about it; she discovered the damage to the car the next time she went out. The car had our business logo on it, so she had to drive around the Hunter Valley to work commitments in a vehicle that was virtually advertising my lack of awareness.

Three months later, early one morning I was preparing to drive to Muswellbrook to pick up some hay for my friend who had a farm. I did it fairly often to help him out. Nothing was unusual or irregular about it.

I reversed out of our driveway and backed straight into a tree on the opposite side of the road. I didn't hear the warning beep-beep-beep that the car's sensor must have been giving out. I do remember that I was programming my destination into the Maps app on the car computer. For no reason, I just kept reversing while I was doing this. It was absent-mindedness, but on a way bigger scale than the usual type of thing that affects people. I was lost in what I was doing.

I got out and checked the back of the car, but—exacerbating my loss of concentration from causing the accident—I detected no damage. When I arrived in Muswellbrook, I saw that I'd hit the tree so hard that the car would need its whole rear end replaced.

Two years later, and with a diagnosis of my condition, I understand that this loss of spatial awareness is common for people who have my kind of brain trauma. I bump into doorways; I knock my knees, shoulders, hips and head against furniture; and I end almost every day with unexplained cuts on my hands and limbs. One day I asked Frankie, 'What's this blood doing on the floor?' We checked Joey and Summer, and they were fine. We inspected my body and found that I had blood running down my shin and didn't know it. *How did I do that?* The blood was dry, so it had been there for a while. My pain threshold has always been very high. I could hurt myself and not know. But this was more than that. In addition to being unable to walk anywhere without bumping into things quite hard, my brain was not sending me a signal that I had been hurt or had knocked something over. It's a scary thing to wrap your head around.

But when it comes to losing control of my body, spatial awareness was minor compared with the humiliation of becoming incontinent.

14

FRANKIE

Stumbling around in the Dark

2019

I came into our bedroom one morning, after Michael had gone back to bed, and found him stripping the sheets. 'What are you doing?' I asked. 'I changed the sheets a couple of days ago.'

Michael might have wanted to change the sheets without me knowing about it, but now I'd caught him in the act, he wasn't going to pretend.

'This is really embarrassing,' he said. 'But I've wet the bed.'

I suppose the amazing thing was, looking back, that we didn't go to a doctor about it that very day. I thought it was odd and disturbing, but we just cleaned up and went on with our life.

Then it kept happening. Michael was going to the toilet every half an hour to relieve himself during the day, and he was getting out of bed to go to the toilet every hour or so during the night. He needed to rehydrate a lot after labouring or exercising, but this wasn't normal, was it? Or *was* it?

Other things began to happen, or they had been happening for a while but were now occurring with such frequency that we couldn't deny there was a pattern. Michael would get up in the night and go wandering—at least I thought he was wandering—but what was happening was that he would get out of bed, go to the bathroom, and go back into a different room before wondering where he was and being uncertain about how to find his way back to our room. Everyone can get a bit confused after waking from a heavy sleep, but Michael was not sleeping heavily and this was happening more and more frequently.

There was also the safety of our young family to consider. One day, I took Summer to her swimming lesson. When I arrived back home, Michael complained about an awful smell in the house. He had opened the windows and was searching for the source. I said, 'When did it start?'

'A couple of hours ago,' Michael replied.

After investigating for a while longer, we found that the gas was on. Michael had turned on one of the stovetop burners to cook something, but he hadn't lit it or turned it off. He'd just forgotten all about it. A couple of days later, he had no memory of that incident, and he did it again.

His balance was off, like a person with a physical disability. He would get up during the night to make yet another trip to the toilet, and I'd hear a crash as he fell over and hit the floor. Once he lost his balance and nearly smashed through the shower screen. Night-time became a source of unending worry to me, as I didn't know where Michael would end up or what damage he would do to himself. I would go looking for him, and his eyes would be glazed over; he would barely recognise me. The next morning, he would be irritable and frustrated with his concentration lapses and loss of memory. He was never aggressive—just exasperated with himself and others—and, of course, he was embarrassed by what had gone on during the night.

The wandering and the incontinence were frightening for both of us, of course, but in real life you don't sit around with your teeth chattering and saying how scared you are. In real life you cover up your fear by arguing or disappearing or being unreliable and antisocial. Sometimes I thought Michael was acting like a big fat arsehole. But it wasn't until later that doctors told us the night-time events were a kind of seizure associated with traumatic brain injury, and the incontinence was a dysfunction called neurogenic bladder, which is common among people whose brains aren't relaying the right messages to their bladder. When it's put that way, it all makes sense. But that was still way ahead of us. We were still stumbling around blindly in the darkness—literally.

15

MICHAEL

The D-word

2019–2020

I received a message via Instagram from someone called Alix Popham. He had founded an organisation called Head for Change, a charity directed at sportspeople who had suffered from concussion. Alix's message said he had information that I had endured more than 30 concussions during my career. Did I want to hear more about Head for Change?

It took me a month to get back to him, and I wrote, 'Sorry, do I know you? Are you a reporter? A fan?'

Alix sent me a link to his biography. Of course, I knew him! He was the same age as me, he had played 33 times for Wales, and he had a thirteen-year professional career—from 1998 to 2011—virtually the same period as me. I always really liked him and *loved* the way he played, a courageous man who threw himself into the fray without a care about his body. I admired him; he was also a back rower, and a player in the same mould as me. He had blond hair that went everywhere as he flew into head clashes. He was incredibly robust for all the punishment he put himself through.

But I'd completely forgotten him . . . which answered his question about whether or not I was suffering from the after-effects of my career.

I apologised to Alix and said yes, I would like to learn more. He told me about his charity, and mentioned what was being done in terms of a class action against World Rugby (formerly known as the International Rugby Board), the governing body for the code of rugby union around the world. Questions had been raised about whether World Rugby could and should have done more to protect rugby players, many of whom suffered serious brain injuries during their playing days and had to deal with the consequences for the rest of their lives.

He let me know that the concussion issue had become a big deal with the National Football League (NFL) in the United States only when the organisation had begun to feel the financial pressure of being sued. The information had been out there for a long time, particularly after the class action by former NFL players, but rugby hadn't treated it as urgently. A possible law suit in rugby might bring similar legal pressure to bear on World Rugby, to get justice for retired players and guarantees of safety for those playing now and in the future.

Alix put me and Frankie in touch with Richard Boardman, the solicitor acting on the players' behalf in this class action.

Richard said to me, 'We know a bit about your concussion history, as it's been extremely well-documented on the internet. Have you been going through the following things?' He listed symptom after symptom: memory loss, concentration failures, balance issues and physical problems such as incontinence.

Frankie was by my side during this call. We looked at each other and said, 'Yes! Yes! Yes! This is exactly what we've been going through for years!'

It was a magical and liberating moment. It felt like we were being given the key that would unlock the mysterious box that my head and personality had become. We had been struggling with it for so long, every day, not knowing what *it* was. We were almost celebrating that others were going through the same terrible experiences as me.

Richard said that we needed a neuropsychological assessment and another brain scan. He knew someone in Melbourne who could do a more specific kind of scan for me. 'In the United Kingdom,' he said, 'you've normally got to be part of a university research project to get this scan. It's how they see if you have that protein build-up in your brain that points to CTE. You can't see that in a regular MRI.'

This was the first time we heard those initials: CTE (the abbreviation of chronic traumatic encephalopathy). CTE was still in the very early stages of being understood, in part due to the fact that it can only be certifiably diagnosed in autopsy: that is, you can only tell if a brain has been damaged by the repeated head trauma that results in CTE when that brain has been removed from a dead person. But everything in my list of symptoms pointed towards probable CTE. I was floored, yet at the same time was flooded with relief.

Richard and the Head for Change group put us in touch with Macquarie University's Dr Rowena Mobbs, an Australian leader in the study of dementia: the dreaded D-word. I had to do more testing to see if my symptoms consolidated into an actual diagnosis. I was only 40 years old; even to say the D-word, and to be recommended for dementia testing, was confronting to say the least. But the time had arrived when my need to seek answers had finally overcome my desire to run and hide from what was happening to me, or to be the big man and pretend all was well.

In 2020, I met Dr Mobbs for a consultation and to do a number of cognitive tests and an EEG (electroencephalogram). She made notes about my condition, and here is what she wrote:

- Previously a cheerful, easy-going fellow, smart, no issues during childhood.
- In 2016, developed chronic headaches, low mood alongside progressive short-term memory impairment.
- By the time I saw him in mid-2020, this had progressed to longer-term memory loss, worsened mood and behavioural outbursts associated with his distant history of severe concussion and head-injury exposure.
- Cognitive testing confirmed impairments of learning and memory, frontal executive functioning that fits with the history of difficulty multitasking, making decisions,

concentrating and changes of impulsivity, along with other deficits that formed a picture of early-onset dementia.
- This is associated with a decline in regulation of his behaviour and at times heavy drinking, although a relatively new occurrence.
- More significantly, Michael was documented to have suffered around 30 concussions and 21 years of exposure to subconcussion with rugby.
- Investigations such as EEG and MRI found no other causes, and his migraine, mood and behavioural changes have been treated.
- He has continued to experience cognitive impairments despite resolution of his drinking, and the picture is of decline, consistent with probable CTE.

Dr Mobbs sent the test results to the United Kingdom, where they were studied in conjunction with those of the former players who were taking part in the class action. My results were in line with what the doctors were seeing among those players, which gave me mixed feelings. I was reassured that what I was seeing in myself and what Frankie was seeing was real—it wasn't something we were imagining, and I wasn't just being a difficult dickhead—but I also had a grave fear that my symptoms would be the beginning of an irreversible downward spiral.

Allaying this fear was Dr Mobbs's chief contribution, however, and it remains so to this day. Like most people, I thought that if you were diagnosed with early-onset dementia, this automatically meant that you had no hope of stabilising your condition or improving the way you coped with day-to-day situations. I thought that within a few years you would be dribbling and incoherent, unable to communicate with your loved ones, and would require around-the-clock care—basically you'd be a lost cause. That is definitely not true.

Dr Mobbs told me that she specialised in injuries resulting from repetitive head trauma. Thanks to my contact with Alix Popham, Richard Boardman and the Head for Change group in the United Kingdom, I had been put in touch with the perfect doctor for me, just an hour and a half from my home. Dr Mobbs changed my medication and geared it to my symptoms. She told me why things were happening to me, what was going on inside my brain and my body, and where it would lead from here. Being given that understanding by a fantastic communicator set me free.

The consultations with Dr Mobbs led to a meeting with Professor Jennifer Batchelor, a clinical neuropsychologist. She ran a number of further tests on me that changed everything.

The first test involved a series of picture cards. Professor Batchelor said, 'I'm going to hold up a card, and you need to tell me if you've seen this card before.' She dealt them out, and I had to answer yes or no.

Then it was puzzles: I had to put the pieces together within a certain time frame. I found this really hard and arced up. 'I'm not doing it,' I said. 'No!' This was just my ego. I knew that not being able to do a simple puzzle would be humiliating, and I didn't want her to see.

She then asked me a series of questions about Joey, and I got emotional. I think she was reminding me of the big picture, the real reason I was going through this process. Her unspoken message was: *Get over yourself and your ego, Michael—think about what you can do for Joey.*

We got back to the tests. There was problem-solving, maps and 'repeat after me' sentences. I knew that I was going to struggle to repeat what Professor Batchelor had said, and I panicked. To myself I said, 'Okay, okay, just repeat some of the vague details you've retained; you can do it.' But I could not find anything in my head that was even close to what she'd said.

This went on for three hours, just the two of us in a room with all of these blocks and cards and puzzles that were exposing every corner of my incompetence. I was freaking out. I got so frustrated at not being able to do what she was saying, I nearly walked out of the room. By the end, I was exhausted.

Professor Batchelor wrote that my results were so bad, it was almost like I was in an advanced state of psychiatric trauma.

Dr Mobbs also did some memory tests with me, using cards and sentences, but her tests were a lot shorter, only 20–30 minutes as an initial assessment of cognitive impairment. Unlike with Professor Batchelor's tests, I didn't feel like I was doing all that poorly. I thought, *I've done all right here.*

Afterwards, Dr Mobbs gave me a couple of prescriptions, and I left. She compiled a report and sent it to me. I was still in denial. I brushed over it, choosing not to read it carefully.

But when I settled down to face it, the truth was as clear as a bell. Professor Batchelor and another neurologist gave me a definite diagnosis of early-onset dementia, which was a relief after so many years of silent suffering. Now that I knew my diagnosis, I had a better idea of why I was feeling what I was feeling, and I could focus on beating it. Before, I had put all my effort into denying there was anything wrong with me. It was Frankie who had originally noticed the changes during the first couple of years we were together, and Dr Mobbs and Professor Batchelor who now gave me the tools to deal with my situation.

I know there is a lot of fear associated with dementia, but I have a far greater fear of what could have happened had I not been diagnosed. Without Frankie (and others) identifying the changes in me, I know that nothing good would have happened. I would have spiralled out of control. I might have done something that got me into trouble, something that I didn't mean to do. I could have ended up in gaol or homeless. Without an income, and having spent all of my savings, what would I have done if I hadn't had my own little family of Frankie, Summer and Joey to look after? I shudder to think.

I will talk a lot about Dr Mobbs from here on because her work has such wide and urgent relevance to so many other people out there. But for me, Frankie was the one who saved my life.

16

FRANKIE

My Mission

2020

I can't overstate how much I admired Michael for having the courage to go through the diagnostic process. Yes, he had been fighting and denying the symptoms for at least five years, but we have learned about a lot of retired sportsmen who deny the symptoms for decades and, in fact, never try to do anything. They accept terms such as 'punch drunk', they self-medicate with alcohol, and they are lost to themselves. If they're lucky, they have friends who care for them during their long decline. But a lot of them hide behind a tough-guy mask, and conceal their symptoms from themselves and from others. This kind of behaviour seems tough and 'male' on the surface. However, in my view, it's really men like Michael, who take a backward step and submit to reality for the sake of their wife and children, who are strong and brave.

When Michael began seeing Dr Rowena Mobbs and had his diagnostic tests with Professor Jennifer Batchelor, I was just as scared as he was of what they might say. He was in denial: he was still the tough rugby player. To admit something was wrong, and to know he had to see someone about it—even when he had lost his job and his sense of identity because of it—was soul-destroying for him and also for me. Everywhere he walked, his shoulders and head were slumped, like he was ashamed of himself. It broke my heart to see him like that. But I really did believe that whatever the doctors told us could be the beginning of a journey upwards and out of this fix we were in.

Of course, we were terrified of them saying he had brain cancer or dementia. Who wouldn't be? We wanted to know, but we didn't want to know, if that makes sense. But Michael accepted a bigger need: he had a family, and it was imperative for him to do the right thing by us. Everything he was doing, whether he got medical treatment or not, was having an impact on us. Every single day there were moments in his life, little bizarre things, that could be explained if we had a clear diagnosis. They were not about to go away by themselves.

I have a fixer type of personality, and from the day I first understood that all was not well with Michael, I wanted to step in and do everything myself. I could see that day-to-day tasks which would be second nature for anyone else were becoming more and more difficult for Michael. For example, he had a favourite little trick he would perform for the kids that involved clapping his wrists and hands together to make a sound like a horse galloping. The kids were delighted every time he did it for them. But one night, when he went to do this thing that he had been able to pull off ever since he was a child, he just couldn't do it. He slumped. I saw it on his face: something's really wrong again.

'Try it again,' I said. But he'd lost his good mood and went into a funk. I tried everything I could to reassure him, to tell him that it wasn't important. But for Michael, it was another sign that his motor skills were being affected and perhaps could never be recovered. Little things like this were devastating to him; sometimes the smaller they seemed to us, the more soul-destroying they were for Michael. My role was first to try to fix the situation and not let it spiral into a great catastrophe for him or for us. My next step was to help him accept that easy things becoming hard is just a natural part of ageing, and we all have to deal with it one day.

When it came to seeing Dr Mobbs and Professor Batchelor, it's not like Michael instantly accepted his diagnosis. It was a long work in progress. At first, he didn't want to know. He would come home from an appointment with Dr Mobbs and I would ask, 'So have you read the fact sheets she's given you?' Michael would bluff away before revealing that he hadn't given them a single look. I didn't push him, but instead dived into them myself, digesting all the information I could get. For him it was too confronting at first, but for me it was another fixing job I needed to do.

What was most confronting for me, personally, was when Dr Mobbs made notes about our family situation and wrote that I was Michael's 'carer'. That was a shock. *Oh my goodness,* I thought, *we're in a relationship but that's what I am.* For a long time, we had joked that Michael was my third child, but to see that word 'carer' written down by a doctor was intense for me.

I wasn't so confronted when the diagnosis from the doctors was early-onset dementia and probable CTE. They studied all the variables and ruled out everything else. I had seen the film *Concussion*, and I knew that what Michael had was not the dementia seen in Alzheimer's disease and the other kinds of degenerative brain diseases that usually affect older people. Instead, I reasoned, it was a disease relating specifically to concussion. They could call it dementia, but surely it's not the same for Michael as it is for an old person? I buried my head in books to do all the research I could. For me, this was Michael, the husband I love, not a medical case—and certainly not an old man in an Alzheimer's ward.

Once we had the diagnosis, I didn't need a second opinion. CTE explained Michael to a tee. The tension in me was released; I wasn't imagining things. He wasn't acting erratically because he was an unreliable or unloving individual. Even though the diagnosis scared the hell out of me, it also gave me a sense of relief. There was a reason all of these things had happened. They couldn't be blamed on his personality or his choices. I was right when I'd stuck to my opinion that Michael is a good person.

Michael didn't share my relief at first, and he still fought against the idea that there was something permanently broken. In his head, he wanted to be that guy who could do anything. And why shouldn't he? He had only just turned 40. I wouldn't want him to passively accept that he was descending into irreversible decline and disability. That didn't mean we sat there and dealt with each other's reactions in peace. We argued a lot. But we also accepted a lot, thanks to the official diagnosis. In time, for example, Michael stopped fighting the fact that he couldn't order food in a restaurant—he just couldn't keep things in his head for long enough or come out with the right words when he felt that he was under pressure from a waitperson—so it became our routine that I would order for him. It's no embarrassment for him; lots of couples do it that way. It's just one of those things that we can explain by his diagnosis. It's not a bad thing. It just is.

I am convinced that getting the diagnosis and other help from experienced and well-intentioned doctors was genuinely a new beginning for us. From that moment on, I stopped wondering about the unknown factors that were making Michael do some strange things. Instead, I gave myself a mission. I started thinking: *What can we do going forward?*

17

FRANKIE

What is inside Michael's Head?

Dr Rowena Mobbs and Professor Jennifer Batchelor had given Michael not just a clear diagnosis, but the beginning of a strategy on how to treat it. But what did 'dementia' and 'probable CTE' really mean? At the beginning, they were just words to us—words that Michael was quick, initially, to reject.

My approach was the opposite. I am one of life's born students. If I want to know about something, I won't stop until I have hoovered up everything I can to improve my understanding. It's not just for interest's sake. Knowledge really is power, and if we were going to gain some power over this disease Michael was suffering from, we needed a lot more knowledge. I thank many people, most of all Dr Mobbs, for guiding my reading in a direction that led to an understanding of the whole history of concussion in sport and where we are up to today. What follows is a digest of everything they steered me towards and everything I have been able to learn about this disease, for the benefit of Michael, myself, Summer and Joey.

Where to start? Probably the best place is the United States, where the science and the politics of concussion in sport collided earlier than anywhere else, and where the most dramatic incidents led to greater urgency in doing something about this scourge.

An American pathologist named Dr Harrison Martland first wrote about 'punch-drunk syndrome' in the 1920s. Concussion had been thought of as a temporary state, even when it brought on amnesia, which was not reckoned to leave the brain with a permanent or structural injury. In 1928, Dr Martland performed autopsies on 309 people who had died from head injuries and found that successive small bleeds, or 'microhaemorrhages', caused permanent damage to brain tissue. Looking specifically at boxers and titling his landmark paper 'Punch Drunk', Dr Martland described the signs and symptoms as a wobbly (or 'Parkinsonian') gait, vertigo and shakiness, and in some cases mental deterioration that was so severe that boxers and other head-injury victims had ended up in asylums. He focused particularly on boxers known as 'sluggers' for their ability to absorb a lot of hits to the head while waiting to land a knockout blow. More agile, evasive boxers who avoided getting hit so much were not as affected by punch-drunk syndrome. It was almost exclusively taking place in the brains of those who were known for their 'courage' in continuing to fight while dazed from the punishment they had taken.

It seems pretty obvious now—we all saw what happened to Muhammad Ali. But until Dr Martland's work, the medical profession did not acknowledge punch-drunk syndrome or any permanent ongoing effects from repeated concussions. When boxers went to medical specialists to seek help, they were actually turned away. Dr Martland learned more from boxers themselves and their coaches, promoters and trainers than he did from other doctors.

A decade after Dr Martland's work, a US naval medical officer named J.A. Millspaugh studied boxers who'd fought in naval competitions, and he came up with a new name for punch-drunk syndrome. He called it 'dementia pugilistica', and the term is still used today for boxers who suffer permanent disorientation and dementia.

Boxing had been around for centuries, so there was plenty of evidence by then. The sport itself had recognised the problem when it introduced its 'Queensberry rules' in the nineteenth century to stop unlimited savagery, such as boxers kicking and punching their opponents when they were already unconscious on the ground. After Millspaugh's study, further rules were brought in to stop fights when one of the boxers became visibly groggy. But even in a sport that was so obviously harmful for these men, humans sure took their time in doing something about it. It took until 1979 before the New York boxing authorities allowed a doctor to intervene and stop a fight where the losing boxer was being beaten senseless.

Sometimes it was left to the women. In the 1950s, a British neurologist named Macdonald Critchley wrote about 'the story of the boxer who eventually gives up the ring, having failed to make the grade, later to become what they call a "punch-bag"—that is, one of a team of sparring partners who helps a first-class heavyweight to train. A typical story was that the [punch-bag] boxer, after a promising early career in the ring, begins to slow up; to be knocked out more often; to win fewer contests; and to be seedy for increasingly longer periods after each affray. Most characteristic of all is the admission on the part of the boxer that he finally abandoned the ring because of his wife's increasing disapproval of his career.' Few in boxing really paid attention to the wives, though.

Critchley also used the term 'chronic traumatic encephalopathy', which had been coined in the 1940s to describe psychiatric states found in adults and children who had been subjected to repeated mild head injuries. This would be very important, as Critchley was studying not so much the severity of the injuries as their number and repetition. His main interest was in the dementia-like effects that arose from long-term, repeated, 'minor' damage rather than the issues caused by a single yet spectacular knockout.

The term 'chronic traumatic encephalopathy' did not catch on, however. It fell into disuse for almost half a century. There were more studies of punch-drunk boxers as the evidence mounted up. In 1973, another American pathologist, J.A.N. Corsellis, studied the brains of fifteen dead boxers and found a correlation between the symptoms of dementia pugilistica they had suffered while they were alive and the signs of bleeding, scarring and other deterioration in their brains. These same brains were preserved and re-examined in the 1990s, when new techniques found further markers of the specific damage that Dr Martland had described back in the 1920s.

It's pretty incredible to me that the only sport that was a focus for this kind of medical scrutiny was boxing. I know that football codes were much more recently invented, but people had been playing rugby, American football, soccer, rugby league and Australian rules for decades while this significant research into boxing was going on. It's like there was a silent agreement among punch-drunk retired footballers just to accept that they were in a similar state to boxers, but not to mention it. All to do with being a tough guy, I guess.

The resistance to uncovering the extent of brain trauma in the football codes was shown dramatically in *Concussion*, which I watched with Michael, the film that chronicles the experience of neuropathologist Dr Bennet Omalu. It was Dr Omalu who rebirthed the term 'chronic traumatic encephalopathy' (shortened to CTE) and changed the understanding of football-induced concussive injuries.

In 2002, Dr Omalu went to work in his Pittsburgh lab to do an autopsy on 'Iron' Mike Webster, an NFL footballer who had died at the age of 50 from a heart attack. Webster had been a hero of the Pittsburgh Steelers team that won four Super Bowls in the 1970s. Webster's position was centre—the so-called 'tip of the arrow'—the huge strong guy who stands in the middle of the offensive line, 'snaps' the ball between his legs to the quarterback and then absorbs someone equally huge charging at him as he tries to protect his precious playmaker. Webster played twenty seasons of college and professional football in this position and was one of the all-time greats, being chosen as centre when the NFL named its best-ever teams on the 75th and 100th anniversaries of American football.

But in the twelve years after his 1990 retirement, Webster's life had progressed on a terrifying downward spiral. He was visibly 'punch drunk', and he had lost all of his possessions. In his last few years, this poor man had been living in a ute with its windows replaced by taped-up garbage bags, sniffing glue (and putting his broken teeth back together with Super Glue), and anaesthetising himself with a taser gun to deal with his body pains and also, in the end, just to get to sleep. His behaviour had become increasingly bizarre over the years, with disappearances and memory loss, paranoia and explosive reactions affecting all of his relationships with friends and family. He had given away or lost all the money he made from football.

Webster's heart had failed, causing his death, but Dr Omalu was more interested in his brain. He wanted to know what was behind the behaviour leading up to Webster's end, and he had his suspicions about dementia pugilistica. He had also examined the brains of motorcyclists who had died in accidents. Their heads were completely unmarked by any outward physical injury but their brains, having rattled around inside their helmeted skulls, were in a damaged state.

CT and MRI scans of Webster's brain were clear. There were no obvious bleeds or scars on the surface. There was none of the shrinkage you would see with Alzheimer's disease. Dr Omalu got permission from Webster's family and the go-ahead from his boss to examine the brain over a long period, slicing up sections to dye and put on slides, working late at nights and even taking the brain home with him. He believed that he was hearing Webster calling out from beyond the grave, asking him to help.

Finally, Dr Omalu saw the answer under his microscope. Examining the sections of Webster's brain, he saw 'Brown and red splotches. All over the place. Large accumulations of tau proteins,' according to Jeanne Marie Laskas's groundbreaking *GQ* magazine article, on which the movie was based. 'Tau was kind of like sludge, clogging up the works, killing cells in regions responsible for mood, emotions, and executive functioning. This was why Mike Webster was crazy.'

Dr Omalu and his boss were seeing the visible evidence of a disease that researchers going back to Dr Harrison Martland had inferred from their autopsies. New technology helped Dr Omalu give a new definition to the old term chronic traumatic encephalopathy.

Naively thinking that the NFL would be grateful to understand what exactly was happening to its retired players, Dr Omalu published his findings in the medical journal

Neurosurgery. Regarding the sport's reaction, he was well wide of the mark. He told Laskas, 'There are times I wish I never looked at Mike Webster's brain. It has dragged me into worldly affairs I do not want to be associated with. Human meanness, wickedness, and selfishness. People trying to cover up, to control how information is released. I started this not knowing I was walking into a minefield. That is my only regret.'

The football industry had turned against Mike Webster even while he was still alive. Webster had applied for a disability pension from the NFL, with four doctors verifying that he had a 'closed head injury resulting from multiple concussions'. They estimated that during his career, Webster had been hit by the equivalent force of a car collision more than 25,000 times. The NFL gave him the lowest level of compensation, a pension of US$3000 a month. He died while waiting for a court appeal against what Laskas called 'a multibillion-dollar entertainment industry that seemed to have used him, allowed him to become destroyed, and then threw him away like a rotten piece of meat'.

The NFL did have their Mild Traumatic Brain Injury Committee, but they rubbished Dr Omalu's published paper and demanded that he and the journal retract it. None of the four doctors on that committee was a brain specialist, though, and its chairman was a rheumatologist. Dr Omalu did not back down. Instead, he doubled down, writing about another NFL player he examined soon after Webster. Terry Long had died at the age of 45 after drinking antifreeze.

Like Webster, he had suffered memory loss and episodes of strange behaviour; he had become homeless and attempted suicide several times. Dr Omalu found the same accumulation of tau protein in Long's brain as he had found in Webster's. 'This stuff should not be in the brain of a 45-year-old man,' he said. 'This looks more like a 90-year-old brain with advanced Alzheimer's.'

Dr Omalu wrote another *Neurosurgery* paper and was again pressured and denounced by the NFL. A reporter, who visited Dr Omalu's house and saw the Webster and Long brains sitting there, warned him that someone connected with the NFL might steal the brains and kill him to destroy the evidence.

In time, someone who was connected with the NFL did believe Dr Omalu. Dr Julian Bailes, a neurosurgeon who had worked as a team doctor for the Pittsburgh Steelers, offered Dr Omalu his support. He had been wondering for years about the link between football and what he had seen happening to his friend, Mike Webster, to Terry Long and to others. Their work together led to Dr Omalu examining the brains of more NFL footballers after they died in horrifying circumstances. Former Philadelphia Eagles player Andre Waters shot himself in the mouth in 2006. Dr Omalu found the same CTE in Waters' brain as he had found in Webster's and Long's. Same with Justin Strzelczyk, a 36-year-old retired Steeler who drove his car into an oncoming petrol tanker in 2004. Tom McHale, a former Tampa Bay Buccaneers player who died at 45 after a drug overdose following a long decline into dementia-like behaviour, was another player in whose brain Omalu found CTE. By 2009, Dr Omalu had uncovered fifteen separate cases.

As Cyndy Feasel wrote in her tragic book about her late husband, Grant, entitled *After the Cheering Stops*, the suicides were only the tip of the iceberg, 'since a vast majority of former players do not take their lives with their own hand but instead prematurely die for other reasons—such as heart failure, cancer, Alzheimer's disease, dementia, or end-stage liver disease'.

By 2007, five years after Dr Omalu had alerted it to the Mike Webster case, the NFL was beginning to wake up. It started its own long-term study of the effects of concussion on 120 retired players. This took five years to complete, and only sometime after it was underway did the NFL begin to bring in concussion protocols for current games. 'Medical decisions must always override competitive considerations,' it finally acknowledged. Then, Sylvia Mackey, the wife of a former player whose life, she said, had become a 'deteriorating, ugly, caregiver-killing, degenerative, brain-destroying tragic horror', forced the NFL to increase its financial compensation to ex-players suffering dementia.

More and more NFL players were donating their brains to the VA-BU-CLF Brain Bank at Boston University, which examined them post-mortem. By 2015, the Brain Bank was coming up with conclusive results: 96 per cent of the brains of former NFL players donated to the bank showed CTE, and out of all the footballers' brains donated (this included college and high-school players), 79 per cent showed signs of CTE. Dr Ann McKee, one of the leaders of this project, wrote, 'People think that we're blowing this out of proportion, that [CTE] is a very rare disease and that we're sensationalizing it. My response is that from where I sit, this is a very real disease. We have no problem identifying it in hundreds of [football] players.'

But the resistance to the actual science was still strong. Dr Omalu suffered continued attacks on his credibility from NFL doctors, and many other studies showing dementia among former football players were dismissed. The University of Oklahoma did a study showing how helmets not only failed to protect the brain from the G-forces in concussions and the injuries caused by the rotation of the brain on impact, but actually made such injuries worse, as helmeted players led with their heads into collisions, and the leverage of the faceguard on a helmet caused increased rotational force. They recognised that the most lasting damage from concussions is not from a direct impact itself, but from the twisting and bouncing of the brain—as it floats in its cerebrospinal fluid—when the body or head undergoes an extreme and sudden change of direction. It's the way the brain bounces around in the skull and injures itself against the inside of the cranium that does the damage in concussions. That's why so many victims show no outward injuries or signs of what has gone on inside.

It was maddening for these scientists to be ignored, but the NFL was only giving public credibility to studies that it sponsored, and, of course, its studies were not as damning as those performed by independent experts. Dr Bailes told Laskas, 'Here we have a multibillion-dollar industry. Where does their responsibility begin? Say you're a kid and you sign up to play football. You realise you can blow out your knee, you can even break your neck and become paralysed. Those are all known risks. But you don't sign up to become a brain-damaged young adult. The NFL should be leading the world in figuring this out, acknowledging the risk. They should be *thanking* us for bringing them this research. Where does their responsibility begin?'

Belatedly, the NFL made some minor changes to its rules and brought in a 'concussion protocol' that required spotters watching the game from the press box to bring off players who showed any of seven signs of concussion: loss of consciousness, slowness to get up after a hit to the head, stumbling or tripping over, having a blank or vacant look, being disorientated on the field, clutching their head after contact, or having a visible facial injury. It was a start in looking after players after they had been concussed, but it didn't do anything about preventing concussions in the first place. And it only mobilised the resistance, within the game, from those who were still wedded to the spectacle of 'big hits'. When the NFL announced in 2011 that it would fine and suspend players guilty of reckless head shots, a discussion board showed posts such as: 'This is not good. Freaking women organs running this league'; 'The NFL is turning into a touch football "Nancy Boy" League. Steer your kids that have talent into baseball, basketball or any other sport that will still have dignity left in 2 years . . .'; and 'The pussyification of the NFL continues. Every single goddam year the rules get more and more VAGINIZED.' On TV, broadcaster Stuart Scott said that if such rules were brought in, the game would not be football anymore.

When I read about all of this, it made me so angry I could have cried. In 2002, when Dr Omalu first alerted the football world to CTE, Michael was just setting out on his professional rugby career. By 2009, when the NFL was *beginning* to take Dr Omalu's work seriously enough to bring in concussion protocols and 'satisfy itself' as to the evidence, Michael was still in the prime of his career but getting concussed more and more easily. By 2012, when Michael had to retire, ten years had passed and the NFL was just getting serious about concussion. It wasn't until 2015 that a set of criteria for accurately diagnosing CTE was published; but remember, CTE can only be discovered for sure in an autopsy. It took until 2016 for the diagnostic criteria for 'probable CTE', that is, the clinical symptoms of living people, to be published. The sporting world was only then making a concerted effort to catch up with the science it had been denying. By that time, Michael and I had met, but he was already fighting against the effects of CTE.

It breaks my heart that Michael's entire professional rugby career took place in the exact period when American doctors were alerting the world to CTE in football, and their football code was denying it. And this is just American football. The same damage had to be going on in other football codes. The longer the NFL stonewalled, the longer it took for rugby authorities where Michael played, in Britain and Australia, to do anything about it.

A decade was lost. And that was Michael's decade.

More than 4500 NFL players joined together in a class action against the league in 2012. They made up a staggering one-third of all living former NFL players. Two years later, the NFL agreed to pay them US$765 million in compensation, with a total of US$1 billion allocated to retired players suffering from the effects of head trauma. But the settlement did not acknowledge fault or allow an investigation of the NFL, and more than two-thirds of the claims of ex-players with dementia symptoms were rejected by the NFL's compensation fund.

On the field, there are now 'concussion protocols' and preseason testing, players' cognitive function is monitored before allowing them back on the field, and there are improvements being made to helmets. But the essential brutality of the game is unchanged. Concussions still occur on a daily basis. Former players continue to suffer the effects. The biggest rule changes they made were to adjust the distance of kick-offs and the number of players involved in collisions after kick-offs, which are the part of the game where the speed of players hitting each other is highest. (Note: Mike Webster and those other players mentioned earlier were never involved in kick-offs.) The NFL also regulated heavy contact in training to sixteen days per season, or approximately one session a week.

The NFL has tried to put a bandaid over the problem while preserving the collisions on the field that apparently make this such an entertaining spectacle and Americans' favourite sport—and that generate the billions in revenue.

Because the NFL is so big, and medical and legal resources in the United States are on a greater scale than elsewhere, the rest of the world waited and watched while it struggled with its concussion issue. Only after the NFL acted did the minor American football leagues start to protect children, college players and women players. And only after that did our sports begin to do something. Just as American football spent so long saying dementia from concussions was a boxing problem, our codes spent years saying it was an American football and boxing problem.

It's not as if scientists and doctors weren't aware of the prevalence of concussion in rugby union. Since the 1980s, credible scientific evidence had been published in numerous journals, and it suggested that concussion was the most common injury in rugby in Britain, Australia, New Zealand and South Africa. Most of these studies were of schoolboy competitions, and most of the concern was directed at how to protect younger players whose brains were not fully grown. Padded headgear was already common in rugby from its early times, but concussion was not fully understood then. As with American football players, rugby players thought that padding on the outside of the head would prevent head injuries; what they didn't realise was the impact on the brain when the head suddenly changed direction or was hit hard. Padded headgear would do as little to prevent those concussions as helmets had done for American footballers. If anything, headgear and helmets gave players a false sense of security. Just ask Michael, who wore headgear for almost his entire career.

It was in the United States, ironically, that a little-reported review of rugby concussions was carried out in 2001. The authors, Stephen Marshall and Richard Spencer, wrote, 'Concussion is of particular concern in rugby. Participants are largely unshielded from collision forces, and the cranium is subjected to violent acceleration-deceleration and rotational forces . . . The incidence of concussion in rugby is probably much higher than previously suggested.' In the small sample they studied in a rugby competition in Utah, they found that if a player participated in an entire rugby season, he had an 11 per cent chance of sustaining a concussion. It was easily the most common injury, accounting for 25 per cent of all rugby injuries.

But even then—and this was the really worrying part of their study—they said that the incidence of concussion in rugby was almost certainly underreported by a large factor. The reporting of concussions in school rugby in Utah, they said, was *100 times* greater than the reporting in Australia. This could have been a result of American rugby players coming from a gridiron background and doing more shoulder charges in their tackling, and therefore getting concussed more often, but the authors doubted it. More likely, they said, 'much of the world's rugby is played in situations in which medical personnel are frequently not present. Those medical personnel who are available are often not well trained in recognising and managing concussions. An administrative barrier also affects concussion identification and management. Under the rules of the game, as promulgated by the International Rugby Board, any player who self-reports or is diagnosed as having a concussion is subject to an automatic 3-week suspension from all competitions and team practices. This mandatory 3-week "stand-down" period is supposed to apply even when a player sustains a very mild injury and returns to a normal level of functioning within minutes. As a result of these factors, we came to suspect that many rugby concussions go unreported.'

As Michael could tell you, they did have 'concussion protocols' in professional rugby union while he was playing, and earlier. Since the 1970s, in some rugby jurisdictions there was a mandatory three-week stand-down period after concussions. Bill Beaumont, the England second rower who later became the chairman of World Rugby, retired after several concussions at the age of 29, and that was back in 1982. But this was voluntary. The 'rules' protecting players from the effects of concussions, or those that existed, were easy to get around and many teams and players simply chose not to follow them. It went against all of their rugby instincts and ideas of teamwork to miss games due to concussion. Michael spent most of his career getting up after concussions, shaking himself off and continuing with the game. And he was applauded for his 'courage' in doing so. A study in 2015 found that 75 per cent of British rugby players would continue an important game even if they knew that they were concussed: that is, three-quarters of the players out there were just like Michael. The important thing here wasn't just that they didn't look after themselves; it was that no rugby authority took responsibility for educating players and coaches, or making them aware of the evidence that was already out there. Michael and others simply didn't know what they were getting themselves into.

Only towards the end of Michael's career were concussions being reported more honestly. The year 2011 was the first in which concussions accounted for the highest number of injuries in Premiership Rugby, where he had played for almost a decade for Bristol and Bath. Did anyone seriously believe that concussions suddenly began happening more often in 2011 than in earlier years? Ever since then, concussion has been the most-reported injury in Premiership Rugby. The latest figures show that if a player completes a full season, he has more than a 50 per cent chance of suffering at least one concussion in that time. It sounds like they were getting closer to the truth.

Throughout Michael's career, and even since, the willingness to treat concussion with due seriousness has been questionable. While he was playing, a sideline assessment protocol—the Pitch-side Suspected Concussion Assessment (PSCA)—was performed if a player had suffered a suspected concussion. In 2013, Scottish international Rory Lamont said publicly what all players knew privately: 'The problem with the PSCA is a concussed player can pass the assessment. I know from firsthand experience it can be quite ineffective in deciding if a player is concussed. It is argued that allowing the five-minute assessment is better than zero minutes but it is not as clear-cut as one might hope. Concussion symptoms regularly take ten minutes or longer to actually present. Consequently, the five-minute PSCA may be giving concussed players a licence to return to the field.'

The five-minute break was replaced by the ten-minute 'head bin' at the end of Michael's career, but it was some years before the reliability of the testing was more watertight. It had also been questionable, as it is today, whether trainers employed by the teams to conduct the concussion tests on the players were independent enough. Many trainers wanted to win just as much as the players and coaches. But it is not as if every club in every level of the codes has the resources to have an independent doctor or medical assessor on the sideline of every match. As Michael will tell you, if you leave the decision-making up to the player, he will always do his best to get back on the field, even to his own detriment. The team comes first.

Alix Popham was the high-profile British rugby-union player who broke the mould. Alix represented Wales 33 times and played more than 250 professional matches in the same period when Michael was at his peak. He's only a few months older than Michael, and he was also a back rower who was admired for his fearless tackling and disregard of his personal safety in his heroic feats on the field.

Like Michael, Alix was diagnosed with early-onset dementia. Unlike Michael, among his symptoms he struggled more with outbursts of rage. He said that he broke doors after slamming them so hard, pulled a banister out of the wall in his home, and then, when he was done, he had no idea why he had exploded. His forgetfulness was as bad as Michael's: he once set his kitchen on fire, with his two-year-old daughter in the room, when he forgot that he had put food in his grill, shut the door and turned it on. Alix blacked out during an ordinary neighbourhood bike ride and couldn't find his way home. In groups of people, he lost track of the meanings of words in conversations, and when he was caught not knowing what word to say, he would make up something. His experiences were both marginally different from and totally similar to Michael's.

It is estimated that during his career, Alix suffered more than 100,000 'subconcussions' in full-contact practice sessions and matches. A subconcussion, he said, was like a tap that is dripping onto a stone floor: you don't notice the effect of one, two or even ten or twenty drops, but over the years, if it keeps on dripping, it wears a definite hole. That was what the constant stream of minor impacts, mixed with some major ones, had done to Alix's brain. You don't need a PhD in maths to add it all up. There is no NFL-style mandated limit on heavy contact in training sessions in rugby, even now. Over a ten-month season, elite players with old-school coaches have as many as two to four full-contact sessions in training each week, plus their weekly match.

That can mean they get their head dinged in as many as 200 training sessions and games per season, compared with the 32 to 35 times a season now regulated in the NFL. That is a huge dosage of contact, and it's what players like Michael and Alix did at the top level for more than ten years.

When Alix talked about his international career, it was as sad as hearing Michael talk about his. Alix was in a Welsh team that beat England at Twickenham, and he couldn't remember a single thing about it. He had a photo of himself meeting Nelson Mandela before a Test match in South Africa, but again, he had no recollection. His wife, Mel, and his children had begun to make adjustments so that Alix could take in information, to simplify things enough for him to function—just as we had for Michael. He and his wife were terrified of what state he might be in when his kids were another five, ten or fifteen years older.

After his diagnosis, Alix—whose work following his rugby career had been in the social-media space—went into action. Not only did he go public in order to raise awareness of the dangers of concussion in rugby, but he also joined with Richard Boardman, at the firm Aticus Law's Rylands Sports Law team, to initiate a class action against World Rugby, the game's governing body internationally, and the regional bodies the Rugby Football Union (England) and the Welsh Rugby Union (Wales).

A few months after Alix Popham had reached out to Michael, and once Michael realised Alix wasn't actually a fan or a journalist as he initially thought, but an ex-Welsh international he had respected and admired greatly, he got back to Alix's message that was sitting in his Instagram inbox. (Gotta love that memory of his.) I was then contacted by Mel, Alix's wife, on WhatsApp. Mel asked me when a good time to chat was, and I wanted to speak with her when Michael was out of earshot.

I drove down to my mother's house in Newport and took the call. It was late at night in Australia, sometime in the morning in Wales. From the start we realised that we had many freakish similarities: I was from Newport, New South Wales, while Mel was from Newport in Wales. Her father had also passed away, and she'd had an incredibly strong bond with him, just like I'd had with mine. Like me, Mel had also started her relationship with her husband a while after his rugby career had finished. We were dealing with the worst bits of rugby, without having been there to revel in any of the best bits. I thought I could talk. Well, Mel can talk the hind leg off a donkey. And I say that with the utmost respect and love! The cherry on top of the coincidence cake was that our son, Joey, and their daughter, Darcy, were born a day apart, both with coppery red hair the colour of a shiny new penny.

I paced back and forth through Mum's kitchen and living room, listening to Mel's thick Welsh accent come through the phone. I was not sure whether my mother was listening or not from her bedroom. She was well aware of some sort of trouble, having experienced Michael's behaviour first-hand on more than one occasion.

Mel and I spoke about our husbands' bizarre symptoms and memory blackouts. She opened up about Alix setting fire to the kitchen while their daughter was in her highchair, and then I opened up about Michael leaving Joey in his cot to hop in an Uber and join a dinner at midnight, 40 minutes away. We spoke about manic behaviour, disorientation and arguing. We both cried as we talked about being so desperate for help, desperate to be understood, and to understand, discussing at great length the need for practical help with how to deal with everything. Mel would tell me later that it was the first time she had spoken to someone else who was walking in her shoes, and probably the first time both of us had been honest with another person about what was happening behind the scenes. In her words: 'That first conversation was emotional but reassuring to be able to finally be so open with someone who got it, completely understood the despair, frustrations, fear and helplessness. It gave me strength to know we were in it together—and we would be strong together and help the boys however we could.'

When I questioned her about how she would approach this book that Michael and I were thinking about writing together, given how exposed it would make us, she said, 'Speak your truth, darling girl—all of what you and, more importantly, Michael have been through is because of his brain damage. Let people see the real heartbreak it causes in lives. This is a powerful example to lots of others still suffering or struggling and in denial.'

A beautiful friendship has developed between the four of us, and I am eternally grateful to both Mel and Alix. The support Alix has provided Michael has been overwhelming, and I've never heard Michael open up to someone more easily. They have gone through so much together, and only they can understand what the other is going through, what fears they have for the future.

The Welsh accent gets me giggling, though, every time I hear a singsong voice message come through from Alix. As the comedian Jimmy Carr puts it, 'To put on a good Welsh accent, you just have to sound really confused.'

Mel and Alix are the driving force behind Head for Change, a foundation that pioneers positive change for brain health in sport and supports ex-rugby and soccer players who are affected by neurodegenerative disease as a result of their professional sporting career. They inspired Michael to help do the same thing here in Australia, and along with Dr Rowena Mobbs, Michael founded and began leading the support group called Concussion Connect at Macquarie University.

If Covid hadn't stolen two years of our travelling lives, I am sure we would have found a way to meet Mel and Alix in person by now. I can't wait for the day when we finally get to see our best Welsh friends in the flesh. We even joke that if Joey plays his cards right, Alix might let him date Darcy when they're older. I would love to have the Pophams as in-laws!

Among the nine players who were initially named in the UK suit (Michael being one), another was former England hooker Steve Thompson, one of the stars of their team that came to Australia and won the Rugby World Cup in 2003.

The final was the famous game in which Jonny Wilkinson snapped a field goal to defeat Australia in extra time. But Steve, who won an MBE after that World Cup, remembers nothing of this career highlight. Sometimes he can't even remember his wife's name. Like Michael and Alix, he was diagnosed with early-onset dementia and probable CTE.

Steve's attitude to his rugby career was a bit harsher than Michael's: he said that he would prefer never to have played rather than suffer dementia at age 42, and he did not want his children to play rugby. But the game had been harsh on him. He spoke of the days of full-body-contact training throughout his career that was so tough sometimes he felt too battered and bruised by a week's practice to take the field on the weekend (but he always did). He told *The Guardian*: 'In the old days [getting knocked out] was a bit of a laugh. If someone got whacked in the head, it was: "Oh, look at him, he's had a belt. He'll be up in a minute."'

One of his doctors asked him how many concussions he'd had. Steve asked him back what counted as a concussion. 'Is it when you're totally out?' The doctor told him that wasn't true anymore. So, Steve said, 'Well, I was doing it every training session then, really, when you look at it.' When Steve blacked out during scrummaging drills, his coaches and teammates said he was 'having a little sleep' and he would wake up again soon.

Were the governing bodies responsible? Richard Boardman, with whom we have ended up having a lot of communication since 2020, believes that the situation of responsibility is parallel to what occurred with the NFL and the class action in the United States. Richard said that the risks of concussion were 'known and foreseeable' to the rugby authorities in the 2000s, and they failed the players in 24 ways that he has listed in his correspondence with World Rugby. Alix, Steve, Michael and the rest of the small group at the beginning are part of a much bigger cohort of potential claimants, which now exceeds 175 former rugby-union players in England and Wales, as well as former rugby-league players in a separate lawsuit in England, while actions in France, Ireland and Scotland are in their early stages.

In 2021, they were joined by a bigger and more recognisable rugby name. Carl Hayman was a prop forward in the mighty New Zealand All Blacks team from 2001 to 2007, playing 46 times for his country and 369 professional games in New Zealand, Britain and France between 1998 and 2015. The same age as Michael, Carl was diagnosed with early-onset dementia and probable CTE in 2021.

As a household name around the rugby world, Carl drew more attention to the issue. He has been in regular phone contact with Michael, sharing his experiences and trauma. Carl's family is going through similar problems to ours, as well as issues specific to him. Because Michael came out publicly so early about his diagnosis, even a big fish like Carl looks up to him as a leader of this group.

But, like in the United States, there is always the potential for a backlash. A former All Blacks doctor, John Mayhew, told the media that Carl Hayman's diagnosis of probable CTE and early-onset dementia shouldn't be automatically linked to his 400-plus games of top-level rugby in the middle of the scrum; instead, his dementia might derive from alcohol use and genetic factors. To Richard Boardman, this sounded very much like the NFL's initial reaction, dismissing tens of thousands of collisions on the sporting field as a possible cause for traumatic brain injury (TBI). 'I think the danger is, whenever any sport has a story like this come out, they just focus on their own house,' Richard said in response to Mayhew's comments. 'Well, in reality, this is an epidemic, impacting every contact sport across the world.' In addition to the rugby class action, Richard has also begun representing more than 75 former rugby-league players against their game's authorities.

At the time we are writing this, the rugby-union class action is still in its pre-trial stage, which means it is open for the rugby authorities to make a financial settlement with the former players. The claim states that rugby 'owed them, as individual professional players, a duty to take reasonable care for their safety by establishing and implementing rules in respect of the assessment, diagnosis and treatment of actual or suspected concussive and subconcussive injuries'. Richard believes the evidence is very similar to what happened in the NFL, and the failures of rugby to look after its players were similarly clear. We know that they knew the dangers of concussion long before they did anything about it; when they did bring in protocols, they were not strict in enforcing them at first.

As well as the evidence of common sense, there is research showing that concussions are even more prevalent in rugby than they are in American football. A 2021 study by an independent English body, the Drake Foundation, concluded that 23 per cent of elite rugby players had some brain damage by the age of 25, and more than half of them had suffered some reduction in their brain volume. These were players who took part in a game supposedly protected by head-injury assessment (HIA) protocols. It's scary stuff. But not half as scary as actually living with it. Richard Boardman says, 'Former players struggle with depression, suicidal thoughts, considerable memory loss, violence, aggression, shortness of temper, an inability to concentrate, and incontinence.' He rejects the counter argument that people like Michael, Carl, Steve and Alix knew and accepted the risks they were taking when they started playing. 'It's not about a group action over guys with broken fingers or stiff backs. Guys absolutely accept the risk in terms of broken bones and torn ligaments. But the brain is the brain. Guys don't sign up for permanent brain damage, and not being able to remember their daughter's birthday at the age of 40.'

Among scientists, there is still some debate over the contribution of contact sports to CTE and early-onset dementia. In 2017, an American group led by Dr Jesse Mez of Boston University looked at the donated brains of 202 deceased gridiron players, by far the biggest study yet. Averaged out, these players had had fifteen-year football careers and had died at the age of 67. Before death, they had reported varying degrees of cognitive impairment, mood disorders and other symptoms. Mez's group found that 177 of those 202 brains showed signs of CTE, a massive number.

Because the understanding of CTE is still in its infancy, other scientists had questions for Mez about the study. What is a correct set of criteria for diagnosing CTE? Is it just one accumulation of the tau protein, or a lot? No clear line had been drawn. And what about other behavioural or genetic factors that could have produced the tau protein abnormalities? The history of every one of those 202 deceased footballers was not checked so that alcoholism, other injuries or inherited factors could be positively ruled out. Most of the brains were donated close to death, many of them by men who were also suffering from depression and might have had family histories of psychiatric illnesses. Information about their histories was not consistently gathered. All of these were potentially 'confounding factors' if Mez wanted to draw a straight causative line between repeated head trauma and CTE.

Mez replied that the diagnosis for CTE was the same as the diagnosis for Alzheimer's dementia: a single 'pathognomonic lesion' is enough. It's a bit like cancer. It has different stages, but stage one is still cancer. In any case, Mez said, of the 177 brains in which he had found CTE, only 6 per cent had one or two lesions, while more than three-quarters showed multiple lesions and were the equivalent of stage three and four cancers. There's no such thing as being 'a little bit CTE', and even if there were, the evidence was overwhelming of long-time footballers being 'a lot CTE'.

As for the confounding factors, such as alcoholism and pre-existing psychiatric illnesses, Mez's reply was the scientific equivalent of 'Well, duh . . .' Yes, those footballers with CTE might also have become alcoholics during their lives. Yes, some of them might have already inherited a tendency to psychiatric illness. Yes, in the questionnaires they filled out before they died, they might not have had the clearest recollection of when and how often they had been concussed playing football (because they had bad memories . . .). If the study wanted to be really strict on all of these factors, it did have to allow that repeated concussions might not be the *only* cause of the tau protein abnormalities in those men's brains. But, as Mez wrote, a history of concussions lowered the threshold for the other factors to play out. That is, if you have inherited a predisposition to a psychiatric illness or a proneness to alcoholism, a career of getting banged around in the head makes those diseases far more likely to come out.

Sometimes it frustrated me to read all of this literature. I know that scientists have to be objective and responsible, and follow strict methodologies. But I also feel that those individuals who are suffering the effects in real life, and their partners and families, are well ahead of the doctors and researchers. We know what's happening from first-hand experience, we are going through a daily roller-coaster of the effects, and we see our loved ones suffering in real time, with an alarmingly fast decline. Meanwhile, the scientific community has to get it absolutely right, but this takes them years and years to certify, and then it takes the contact sports where the injuries are incurred years more to respond. During those years, lives are being lost. It breaks my heart. It also means that people like us, at the front line, have to take over the burden of acting right here, right now, to save lives before the authorities catch up with the truth.

What is actually going on inside the brains of Michael and the others that is causing such similar symptoms? Knowledge of CTE is pretty technical, but Dr Mobbs has made it as easy as possible for us to understand, and I have spent the best part of two years researching it.

In the film *Concussion*, the 'wow' moment occurs when the Dr Bennet Omalu character (played by Will Smith) is looking at slides of Mike Webster's brain, which has been dyed to show any unexpected presence of the tau protein. First identified in 1975, the tau protein normally plays a stabilisation role within the neurons in the brain. It helps to regulate memory and habituation, the function of learning things through repeatedly doing them. But in brains affected by Alzheimer's disease, as well as some other forms of dementia and Parkinson's disease, the tau protein is present in abnormal sites. In a brain with CTE, the tau protein shows up in irregular places and at high concentrations.

Dr Omalu likened the build-up of the tau protein in the brain to pouring cement into your plumbing system. It causes all the connections to seize up and blocks off the transmission of normal messages from one part of the brain to another. But because it can't be seen by imaging such as MRI and CT scans, it has to be inferred from symptoms.

Researchers have looked at whether the abnormal spread of the tau protein inside the brain can be caused by anything other than repeated traumatic collisions. A 2015 American study of a brain bank looked at 66 brains that had a documented history of repetitive brain trauma, and 198 brains that did not. Of the 66, there were 21 that showed the tau protein build-up and CTE. Of the 198, not a single one showed the tau protein or CTE.

In Australia, the evidence is just as compelling—and disturbing. Established in 2018, the Australian Sports Brain Bank released its first study in February 2022. Of the 21 brains donated to the bank, more than half—twelve in total—contained signs of CTE. Three of them were from people who had died before they reached the age of 35, and one, in his early fifties, had only played rugby as a teenager. What made it really scary was that six of those twelve had taken their own lives, including high-profile former Australian rules footballers Danny Frawley and Shane Tuck. The doctors at the brain bank said that Tuck's brain showed the worst CTE they had ever seen. The brain of rugby-league legend Steve Folkes, who died from a heart irregularity at age 59, also showed signs of CTE. At the time of writing, around 900 people have now pledged to donate their brains to the Australian Sports Brain Bank.

If you are a non-expert, the medical literature makes your head spin pretty quickly. What I was most interested in were the symptoms for an individual person and details about the progression of the degeneration. What does Michael's future hold? I found out that the list of symptoms was unhappily familiar. Tau protein build-up leads to cognitive impairment, memory loss (both long and short term), loss of inhibition and empathy, loss of spatial awareness, impaired insight, mood swings, and depression and anxiety, to name just a few outcomes. The symptoms are generally divided into two categories: 'thinking-related', which refers to difficulties with memory, concentration, learning, insight and awareness; and 'mood-related', which refers to irritability, depression, anxiety, panic, rage, impulsiveness, loss of empathy and energy, and reduced social activity. When I drilled right down into it, none of this made for happy reading!

According to the Mayo Clinic, CTE as a disease progresses in four stages:

- Stage one: headaches, loss of attention and reduced concentration. (Michael had been going through this for at least two years before we met.)
- Stage two: depression, explosiveness and short-term memory loss. (I would say Michael was well into this stage when we met, but it increased dramatically between 2016 and 2018, with the caveat that, fortunately, he is not an explosively violent or aggressive person.)
- Stage three: decision-making dysfunction and cognitive impairment. (This was also underway before we met, but I noticed a deterioration in our first two years together, particularly when his real estate career was in trouble.)
- Stage four: dementia, word-finding difficulty and aggression. (Certainly, the words are becoming harder for him

to find, but 'dementia' is still a very confronting term for us, and Dr Mobbs says that Michael is still in its very earliest stages. Aggression, off the football field at least, is not part of Michael's nature, and I hope with all my heart that this disease is not going to change him in that way—but the commonness of it in CTE patients does add to our anxiety.)

CTE is certainly preventable, and this is something that had already become Michael's focus when he came out publicly with his diagnosis in 2020. All the medical literature says that it's not a big concussion or a small collection of major head knocks that causes CTE. Instead, it's more likely to be caused by a great number of small concussions and subconcussions over a long period of time. This is why it is more commonly seen in athletes and military personnel who have had repeated exposure to smaller head knocks than in, say, cyclists or motorcyclists who have had one big accident (which is not to say that they don't develop other serious problems). In 2002, for example, the former English football (soccer) player Jeff Astle died with CTE. As far as his family was aware, he had never suffered a major concussion. The damage most likely came from thousands of subconcussive blows from heading the ball in a sport that is less abrasive than rugby.

But the key for us is that if it is caused by something occupational or recreational, such as playing a contact sport, then it is definitely preventable, and if we can contribute one thing to other people's health and wellbeing in the future, it is to help sports administrators and the people who play those sports understand how to avoid TBI.

Prevention for others is becoming a mission in Michael's life, ever since he accepted his diagnosis and commenced his participation in the rugby class action. But for us as a family, the focus is also on treatment and how to help Michael through this difficult time. There is no cure for CTE. But as we have learned in the past two years, Michael's dementia doesn't have to be a steady downward trajectory. The brain can be reshaped, even when it is hampered by the tau protein abnormalities that cause CTE, and a sufferer can do a great deal to learn new things. Habits can be changed.

18

FRANKIE

From Bad to Worse

2020–2021

Jeanne Marie Laskas, who wrote the story of Dr Bennet Omalu's struggle to get the NFL to recognise the link between CTE and concussion from football, wrote a follow-up article in 2011 about retired gridiron player Fred McNeill. Laskas was with McNeill's wife, Tia, as she waited for him one day outside their apartment in Los Angeles. Tia phoned Fred to ask him when he was coming down.

'Am I what?' he replied.

'Are you coming down? I'm waiting.'

'You're waiting?'

'Fred, I'm out here waiting!'

'Oh, okay, I'll come down.'

'Don't forget the suitcase,' she said.

'Suitcase?'

'Remember I need my suitcase back?'

'I don't remember a suitcase.'

'Fred, I just told you ten minutes ago that I am outside waiting for you and to bring me the suitcase,' she said.

'It's too early for karaoke,' he said.

'Coffee. I am taking you out for coffee. Now, come on.'

'Coffee. That sounds good.'

Five minutes later, Fred still hadn't come down, and when Tia phoned him, she was put through to voicemail. It's a maddening scenario, and for me it rang true—it was like I was reading a version of my own life. *People need to know this stuff*, I thought. They need to know so they will treat concussion in sport more seriously, so they will know how to guide their kids on playing contact sports, and so those who are affected by it will benefit from having the same sensation I had when I read about people such as Fred and Tia McNeill: recognition that we are not the only ones.

I was first approached by Peter FitzSimons and Malcolm Knox in January 2021 to talk with the publisher Allen & Unwin about the possibility of writing a book about concussion and how repeated head trauma affects the families of those suffering from it.

Peter had interviewed Michael and me for an online seminar with Dr Rowena Mobbs from the Australian Sports Brain Bank in late 2020, due to his passion for changing concussion protocols in sport. We had agreed to do the seminar as we thought that the only people who would attend would be medical professionals and sports administrators. Peter, a former Wallaby and a well-known author and journalist, had become extremely concerned about the friends and former teammates he knew who were suffering from the after-effects of concussions they'd had while playing rugby. As he investigated, he saw a worldwide change taking place in how sports-induced head trauma was being treated. It had become something of a crusade of Peter's to draw attention to the issue and to get sporting bodies to respond appropriately.

Peter was seriously taken aback when we spoke openly about Michael's cognitive impairment at just 40 years of age. We spoke about the results of Michael's recent tests, and I opened up to Peter about Michael's score on one of his cognitive screenings, the ACE-III (Australian version). When I first read the report, I was naive enough to think that Michael had done well, not understanding that the numbers he had recorded actually meant that he had a mild cognitive impairment and mild dementia. Snippets from a letter that Dr Mobbs sent to Michael's GP still go through my mind: 'reduction in verbal fluency' . . . 'cognitive decline' . . . 'mood disorder' . . . 'mild unkempt nature' . . . 'substance abuse' . . . 'inappropriate at times'. Most resonant of all were three words that I still have problems reading, let alone pronouncing: 'chronic traumatic encephalopathy'.

Michael didn't say much in the interview with Peter, which was totally out of character for him. He normally cannot shut up! But he was withdrawn and reluctant to speak.

We walked out of the seminar room into the foyer, where Peter and Dr Mobbs were sitting down, deep in conversation. Peter looked over at us, and I had the very strong feeling that we were the topic being discussed. They gave us a little wave, and off we went.

A few days later, I received a text message from Peter asking if I could give him a call about a sensitive topic. I was shitting myself. What had we done by agreeing to this seminar? What was he going to publish?

Michael was furious. 'Don't speak with him,' he said.

I called Dr Mobbs. 'What does he want to publish?' I asked.

She advised me to chat with him; he wouldn't write anything without our permission. I found that amazing; my perception of Peter changed in an instant. He showed grace and empathy, and he let us know how important it was to make people aware of the damage concussion could cause. He reassured me that he would respect our decision if we didn't want to have anything published. After days of deliberation, we agreed to let Peter write an article about Michael and the D-word. Dementia at 40.

Several months later, when I met Peter and Malcolm to talk about the book, I knew that Michael would want absolutely nothing to do with it. We were not in the best place in our marriage, and I was too scared to even tell Michael that I went to a meeting without consulting him first, especially considering his illness would be the subject matter. I wasn't even sure we would still be married by the time I put pen to paper, given the levels of chaos and stress in our lives.

Michael hadn't come to terms with his diagnosis of probable CTE and early-onset dementia. He was not really listening to medical advice, let alone anything I said to him. I knew that a book would be out of the question.

I walked into that meeting feeling incredibly nervous. But I was certain that a book was a good idea. It would have helped us if we had read about people in Michael's situation five years earlier than we did, so we could have put a name to what he was suffering from. It might help anyone who is considering playing a contact sport, or parents considering allowing their children to play. But did I want to expose our family and the ugliness of certain experiences? The thought was terrifying.

On the other hand, it was already out there now; we had done a rehearsal for all of this. After Peter broke the ice with his article, Michael and I sat through interview after interview—mostly for UK media outlets—when Michael was in the right mood to discuss the issue publicly. But it became so exhausting and painful for Michael that we asked for a break. One of Michael's symptoms that has worsened quite noticeably in the past two years is his difficulty with speech: stuttering, forgetting words, making clumsy attempts to find the right one. He would become embarrassed, and the more pressure he felt, the worse it became.

Even back in 2014, when Michael appeared as a guest on an episode of SBS's *Insight* program about kids and concussion in sport, he said that he started 'professional-ling' in rugby when he was 21—he was embarrassed by having said that. Making up words would become more and more frequent, and it played a role in ruining his career as a real estate agent. However, Michael is wonderful with the written word. His text messages are perfectly executed and punctuated—especially when he believes that I have done something wrong and wants to express his frustration! But he also writes beautiful and eloquent birthday cards and letters. It's hard to believe that they are written by the same person who can struggle to put words in the right context in conversation. So, if his story were to be told, and if we had a choice between a book and a TV interview, the book would be the preferred method. He would have time to get it right, and he could be working in a medium in which he is at his best.

One of my many concerns was that most books about people with CTE are written after they have died. I am definitely not implying that Michael needed to pass away before we could start a book, but the experiences that would make up these pages were difficult and raw, and I couldn't imagine him wanting to be read about in this light. CTE sufferers who have taken their own lives or died from alcohol-related issues or a drug overdose don't have to worry about what people think about them. We have a family to protect. I had read *After the Cheering Stops* by Cyndy Feasel, her story about her marriage to former NFL player Grant Feasel, who passed away from cirrhosis of the liver and CTE. It struck so close to home that it was frightening. Cyndy told some stories that were actually identical to what I had experienced.

I left the meeting with Peter and Malcolm in tears. I felt guilty for not telling Michael, and my anxiety was at an all-time high. It was a 'no' from me. And a snowflake had a better chance in hell than Michael agreeing to it.

Nine months later, Malcolm got in touch to see how we were going. I put him straight on the phone to Michael. We were travelling better together, and Michael's mindset about a book seemed like it might have changed. But if we were going to do this, it had to be his decision, his narrative. We talked about it at great length and decided that this would be the bravest thing he could ever do . . . and he had been labelled 'too brave for his own good' by journalists and coaches his whole career. His bravery, for better or worse, is what got him here in the first place.

'Why haven't they received the book contract yet?' Michael kept asking as days turned into weeks after he sent it off in the post.

'Did you go through Express Post?' I asked.

'No, just normal mail,' he replied.

I had a sinking feeling that something had been done incorrectly, but I didn't want to question him. It was so common for simple daily tasks to get muddled up and seem almost impossible for Michael to complete. In hindsight, mailing an important contract to our publisher was something I should have overseen.

Sure enough, the contract ended up back in our letterbox, marked 'Return to sender'. Michael had addressed it with no company name, no level, just the building number of the multi-level block in Crows Nest. By this stage, he had already re-sent the contract by Express Post. He did admit that he hadn't put in the specific details that were missing, which explained why the first envelope never got there in the first place.

'I put the contract in the thing . . .' he struggled to say.

'The thing?' I asked.

'Yeah, the letter post thing.'

'Do you mean the envelope?' I asked gently.

'Yup, that's it,' he replied.

When he's struggling with words, I see him searching for them in his head, and sometimes he will say what he thinks is the correct word but is really something quite random: 'decoration' instead of 'detail'; 'improvise' instead of 'elaborate'. He muddles up idioms and expressions so frequently that I can't remember the last time he got one right. Just this morning he said, 'He's worth his pot of gold,' about our signwriter who made a decal for our art studio. 'The apple doesn't fall far from the tree,' he said about someone else. He got that expression right, but he used it in a context that wasn't even remotely correct.

I am ashamed to say that I used to cringe at these little things in public. That combined with his lack of filter would have me quickly kicking him under the table when he was saying something inappropriate. Now we are upfront about it. 'Please give me super clear instructions,' he'll ask when someone wants him to do a task. 'Excuse me if I say something a bit off—I've had head trauma.'

I make part of my living as a voiceover artist, which means that I am highly aware of the spoken word. And the fact that I was a teacher for seven years makes me inclined to correct people's speech (which is a horrible trait). I really have had to practise restraint by just letting Michael say whatever he wants to say. The last thing I want is to embarrass him more than he is already feeling.

However, there are times when I wish I had been around to prevent him from getting into controversial situations. As Michael mentioned earlier, he was given a year's ban at our local family pub for unleashing at a barmaid, something that I didn't know about for a few weeks until I asked Michael why he didn't want us to go there for lunch. I didn't get it. I still don't know if I have the full story because lots of people get into physical altercations and are allowed back in within weeks. Michael apparently called the barmaid a 'fucking moll', which is SO out of character for him. He hates swearing, and he could charm the pants off a snake, especially female snakes. I just couldn't work out why he would lash out like that. Twice he went back to ask if the ban could be lifted. It was a firm 'no' both times.

Another time, we went out to dinner as a family at a local restaurant. We had just started eating when Michael, with a straight face, before asking Summer a question, said, 'We got the funk.' The question was about her meal, so it came out as: 'We got the funk. How is your pizza?'

Summer and I looked at each other with raised eyebrows and back at Michael. 'What?' we both replied.

Summer was giggling away. 'You just said, "We got the funk."'

'No, I didn't. Why the hell would I say that?' He looked really confused, and Summer thought it was a hilarious joke.

I clicked. It was the music. The song 'Who Got the Funk?' was playing in the background, and Michael was answering the chorus line. He wasn't singing—he spoke the words—but he didn't realise that he was, or know why he was doing it, and he didn't believe that he just said them.

I understand why he gets worried about meeting new people and hates small talk. I think the pressure of meeting new people makes him stressed about how he may come across to them, and this stress then makes him waffle or ramble—like he's overcompensating.

After we moved to the Central Coast, we wanted to start a business. We set up a Pinot & Picasso franchise in the Hunter Valley—it's where you can come to learn to paint while socialising with new or old friends, and was successfully operating in studios around Australia. When we were in the setting-up stages, people were coming in and out of the studio to see what we were doing, wanting to talk about the concept and opening date, and so on. Michael was working on the fit-out and must have had many interruptions from people popping in for a stickybeak.

One of our studio neighbours came in and introduced herself to me. She was an artist who owned an art gallery a few doors down from us.

'I met your husband earlier,' she said. 'Is he bipolar?'

Just like that. I couldn't believe it. 'No,' I said, 'he's not bipolar—his behaviour can just seem quite manic at times.'

'Right,' she said. 'I only asked because my father is bipolar, and I can see some similarities.'

This conversation was an eye-opener for me. It made me realise that total strangers were noticing something off about Michael's behaviour. After a situation at a restaurant years ago, when I had first met Michael, my best friend had joked that it seemed like my new boyfriend was on the spectrum. Michael had been getting very impatient about something to do with our seating, and he became a little manic. His levels of frustration were sky high, and we did what had become our little routine. I'd gently squeeze him on the arm or leg and say, 'It's okay. You need to calm down, it's not that bad.' I was constantly answering for his strange behaviours, without knowing the cause.

CTE manifests in different ways in different people. Changes in behaviour and personality would have been easier for me to recognise had I been with Michael longer and realised he was changing. I thought that this was just the way he was.

If you're a caregiver of someone with CTE or any of these neurodegenerative diseases, you must understand that they have a different reality to your reality. Getting angry at someone doesn't help. If someone makes a

> mistake or says something in public that is perhaps not the right thing to say, or they yell—getting angry at them or thinking that they are in control of what they are doing, doesn't do anyone any good. So, what I always tell people is—don't argue. Arguing doesn't make any difference. If someone's brain is unable to deal with things logically or have adequate judgement because the parts of the brain that are responsible for that are hurt, it doesn't make any difference for you to argue logically. Even if an hour ago he was screaming at you, throwing things around the house, those things might not be in his control, and if he's in despair now, give him a hug, give him some hope. Give him some attachment. Give him the tools to get him to the next day.

I found this advice from Robert A. Stern, Professor of Neurology at the Boston University School of Medicine, on a YouTube clip shared on a support page on Facebook. I rewatch it when I need a gentle reminder not to lose my temper at something Michael has done, to just take a deep breath and detach myself. Instead of fighting each other, we need to focus on fighting together against the disease.

By 2021, the stress of what was happening to Michael had begun to affect me physically and mentally. I started to have panic attacks in my car on the freeway. I would be driving up to the Hunter Valley and suddenly I couldn't feel myself performing that function anymore, like my body was not in the car, and some other force was controlling the vehicle.

There were moments of hallucination, and this freaked me out so much that I couldn't breathe properly and had to pull over on the side of the freeway until the tightness in my chest went away. This could sometimes take half an hour. With trucks hurtling past me at 100 kilometres an hour, trying to calm down was near impossible. Once I had returned to semi normal, I couldn't drive any faster than 80 kilometres an hour, gripping the steering wheel so tightly my knuckles turned white.

These attacks happened around six times before I decided to get help. I spend so much time on the freeway between the Hunter and Sydney, it was impossible to keep going like this, and I couldn't bring the panic attacks under control on my own. I thank God I never had the kids in the car while I was undergoing these episodes.

I was put on antidepressants to try to prevent further attacks from happening. When discussing this at our second meeting of Concussion Connect with the partners of the other sufferers, I was told by the neuropsychiatrist who treats Michael that she was surprised I wasn't on antidepressants sooner. It was somewhat consoling to hear.

'Please, all I ask of you is that I'm able to see my son on weekends, as he is the only thing in my life worth living for.'

The text came through a couple of days after Michael had left home. It was just after Valentine's Day 2021, and an argument over him not wanting to spend the day with me had escalated to the point where I told him that I didn't think our marriage would survive.

'Are you throwing me out?' he asked sarcastically. 'Because once I'm gone, I'm not coming back.'

'That's your choice,' I responded.

We had been in a bad way, yet again. I was so sick of arguing. I was tired of the ongoing, always repeating 'Michael Show'. We had just spent three months doing interview after interview with the UK media, where the announcement of the class action was a massive news story. Michael retelling his story over and over again was taking a toll on both of us. On top of that, we were having numerous meetings with the legal team and with British doctors, which always seemed to take place during the kids' 'witching hour'—we were still trying to work out the UK/Australia time difference. I would sit down to a meeting and moments later would have to spring up from my seat to sort out an argument or help with a homework question; we relied on YouTube Kids to babysit while we had very serious conversations over Zoom.

Michael was no longer getting up early in the mornings. Sometimes he wouldn't get up until 11 a.m. When we first met, he was up at 5 a.m. every morning for a 5 kilometre run, and then he would pick up a coffee for me on the way home. Fast-forward to 2021, and I was now the one up at the crack of dawn, taking Summer to swim squad and having to drag a two-year-old along with us because his father had refused to get out of bed to help with the daily routine. I know

now that this was a mix of exhaustion and depression, and Michael wasn't doing this intentionally. It was the disease, but it added to the overwhelming feeling I had that *I was doing everything*. So, when he chose to spend Valentine's Day Sunday with his mates instead of me, and then refused to come home when I needed him, I felt extremely unappreciated. *This is the thanks I get,* I thought.

While I was at work the next day, Michael packed a bag and left. I didn't hear from him for a couple of days, he didn't tell me where he was going, and the next contact I had was this text message telling me that Joey was the only thing that made his life worth living. Moments after receiving that message, I got a call from Joey's day care. One of the teachers told me quite worriedly that Michael had come in, distressed and in tears, asked to see our son, said his 'goodbyes' and left again, leaving Joey absolutely beside himself.

Blood rushed to my head. I called Michael straight away. His phone was switched off. I had visions of him driving off a bridge. *He is the only thing in my life worth living for . . .* the words circled around and around in my head. I was panicking. After a few months of delving into the world of CTE research, I knew that self-harm and suicide featured heavily.

I called Dr Rowena Mobbs in hysterics. 'I think he's going to do something to himself, his phone's off, he said goodbye to Joey in the middle of the day, and I don't know where he is or where he's been for days . . . we had a fight . . .' My voice trailed off. She listened patiently and tried to reassure me.

After a few hours, Dr Mobbs messaged me to tell me that Michael was okay, and he was safe. She had managed to get in contact with him, and he asked her not to tell me anything other than that he was okay. He would have seen the countless messages and pleas from me when he turned on his phone. Relief flooded over me. I just wanted to see his face. He was still ignoring my calls and messages, though, so I took a break from trying to contact him. He was safe; that was all I needed to know.

Another couple of days went by. My phone beeped on the Friday morning: 'Can I come home? I miss my family.'

'Of course,' I replied.

Within a few hours he was back. I had told the kids he was away for our business, so as not to worry them. They squealed with delight as he came through our sliding doors and into the lounge room.

'Yay, Michael's home!' Summer screamed from the top of the stairs. She came running down and launched into one of his classic bear hugs.

I joined the family hug and wet his shirt with my tears. 'I'm so sorry,' I cried.

'Me too,' he said.

Three months later, he went off to his mate's place for the weekend. His phone was off again, and he gave me a line about 'not having a charger' when I questioned him. He walked in through the door on the Monday morning and crawled into our bed. No explanation, no apology. I was desperate for a 'sorry', an acknowledgement that he should have called, but now all he wanted to do was sleep. I don't know what I was expecting; getting an apology from Michael is like drawing blood from a stone. I pressed the issue, and he yelled, 'S. O. R. Y!'

I laughed cruelly at the spelling mistake. It tipped him over the edge, and I'm not prepared to write in detail about what happened next. I want to make very clear that there was no threat to harm me in any way—there never has been—but he screamed out that I made him want to kill himself. What happened next led to me running out through the bedroom door and getting on the phone to Rowena Mobbs, who told me to call the mental health centre at Gosford Hospital. Michael had had the very definition of a manic episode. We needed serious help.

19

MICHAEL

Reaching out for Help

September 2021

In her constant search for information about concussion and the long-term effects of TBI, Frankie had read the book *After the Cheering Stops*. It was written by Cyndy Feasel, the widow of Grant Feasel, an American footballer who had been one of the highest-profile players to lose his life after a long battle with the after-effects of concussion.

Only, Grant Feasel didn't die from concussion or TBI as such. As Cyndy writes at the beginning of the book, 'Grant drank himself to death—a slow, lingering process that took nearly twenty years. He didn't press a gun to his heart and pull the trigger like San Diego Chargers linebacker Junior Seau did, but Grant committed suicide all the same. He drank to dull the pain that began in his brain—a brain muddled by a history of repetitive trauma and symptomatic concussions. He drank and drank . . . until the alcohol killed him.'

When Frankie relayed this to me, it wasn't hard to understand the subtext. In fact, it wasn't subtext at all. We had discussed my alcohol use since the beginning of our relationship.

I had enjoyed a drink since I was a very young man. It is part of the culture of rugby around the world to share the joys of success and the sorrows of defeat with your teammates and your opponents. The camaraderie of rugby, which I believe is more universally shared than in most other sports, is built around the clubhouse bar and the pub. Sure, there are teetotal and abstemious rugby players everywhere, and I have no doubt they enjoy the game as much as everyone else, but I was not one of them. The cycle of training hard, playing hard and then celebrating hard was what rugby was all about for many of us, and I make no apology for that. I was known as a good team man, which can be a euphemism for the first to round up everyone for a trip to the pub and the last to go home when last drinks are called. The fact that I spent so many of my best years playing in England added a cultural element to this. In England, drinking alcohol is a revered national pastime, particularly in the winter months when rugby is played, and I was a very happy participant.

Was I a problem drinker? I don't think so (if you take the TBI out of the equation). But that's the thing: I was trying to take it out of the equation before I had my diagnosis because I didn't know I had it. I thought that the period of excessive drinking in the late stages of my real estate career and the occasional big nights out—with the blackouts and memory lapses that inevitably followed—were examples of simply having too much to drink. Only when I received my diagnosis did I have a way of fitting my alcohol use into a bigger and more complex picture.

Before I started seeing Dr Rowena Mobbs, I had become aware that when I had three or four drinks, I was behaving like I had had ten. And that's a problem. Normally, three drinks means that you're chatty, relaxed, bright and sociable. Ten drinks means that you're tripping on your chair as you get up to go to the bathroom, fumbling with the door lock, holding yourself against the wall to keep your aim steady, and, with luck, finding your way back to your table. You might even be blacking out for periods and acting out of character towards your friends and loved ones. My problem was that I was getting like that very early in the piece, and the number of drinks it took to make me behave that way was shrinking by the year. If I wasn't careful, just one or two drinks would be all it took to have me falling over. And if it came to that, and I was getting behind the wheel of a car knowing I would still register below 0.05 on a breathalyser, who knows where it would have led?

Dr Mobbs was absolutely adamant on the issue. Drinking, she said, amplified all of my symptoms by an incalculable factor. The mood swings, the loss of balance, the irritability, the slurring words, the forgetfulness—all of these things were more frequent and more severe if I had been drinking.

It took me a long time to face up to this because, while it might have been a devil for me, drink was also my friend. At times, it was the first place I would look to if I wanted to feel happy, if I wanted to de-stress, if I wanted to unwind, and if I wanted to forget the troubles that were creeping into every day. My self-esteem was on a downward trend, and drinking helped me to forget myself, in what I thought was a good and welcome way. I really, really didn't want to let that friend go.

I never had the feeling that it was as simple as my symptoms being caused by alcohol. I didn't drink enough for it to be the cause of the dramatic effects I was experiencing, such as the blackouts and the loss of memory, at such a young age. As someone who stopped drinking 35 years ago, Frankie's mother knows about Al-Anon and works as a volunteer at the Northside Clinic in Sydney. She encouraged Frankie to attend Al-Anon meetings and investigate the possible connection between alcohol and what I was going through, although she was certain that it had to be something other than alcohol. She had never seen anyone with 'wet brain', a term for dementia acquired through excessive alcohol consumption, but the consensus was that it was pretty much impossible for someone as young as I was to have developed my symptoms from alcohol use alone.

But that didn't change the fact that drinking wasn't helping me one bit and, even if I could not blame it for my diagnosis, I couldn't ignore it, either. It was not making our lives better in any way. Once I'd had a number of good conversations with Dr Mobbs and Frankie about it, I knew that I had to rub alcohol out of my daily routine. It wasn't a question of whether alcohol was 'to blame' or not. It was just that I could make a real improvement to my life if I stopped drinking. By late 2021, Frankie and I were reeling from crisis after crisis. Our marriage was in definite trouble. As far as my brain injury was concerned, I couldn't make those 30 concussions un-happen. But as far as my drinking went, there was something practical I could do.

In September 2021, we decided to knuckle down and face reality. The best way for me to tackle any problem in life is head-on. That's just my nature. So, with the drinking, I couldn't do it subtly or through small steps. I had to make a huge commitment and do it in a big way, which meant being admitted to the mental health clinic at the Brisbane Waters Private Hospital, with the clear goal of stopping drinking.

My life, when it was at its most productive, had been all about simple goals: be on time, do your job, win games. From boarding school through to professional rugby, from the age of twelve to 32, it was all very structured. That structure had made my daily decisions for me. There were exact times for everything. I felt that having the structure of a mental health clinic, as an inpatient, with timetabled classes and requirements to attend activities at specific times of the day, was going to work for me.

On top of making that commitment, I also needed time and space to myself. Being in the clinic would be the first time in my life I had ever been forced to sit and reflect on myself, reflect on who I am, how I'm perceived, who I'm going to be, what example I'm going to set my kids, how I'm going to support and love my wife. Who am I, really, now that I've been retired from rugby for nearly a decade? I had never allowed myself that time, as I'd always loved to surround myself with other people. I had never even been out for a meal by myself. To go into that clinic and be forced to look at myself in the mirror, and search hard—that's when I realised, *Jesus, I've been making bad decisions for too long.*

I went in on 9 September 2021.

The lead-up to my admission was very hard. One morning, two days before I went to the clinic, I spontaneously broke down in tears while hanging the washing on the line. I was looking at myself placing Joey's and Summer's clothes on the line, knowing that I wouldn't see them for three weeks . . . and it was heartbreaking.

I was a lot better the day after, thanks to multiple discussions with Frankie and my support group. It was sinking in why I was going there. Then, at 2 p.m. on a Thursday afternoon, I finally walked through the doors. My temperature was checked, and I began filling out all of the admission forms. My name was called, and I walked into the ward.

All at once, I started to feel completely overwhelmed. *What am I doing here? How has my life come to this?* I was cracking up with shame. *How can I live without my family for three weeks? What will I do, and how am I going to get through it? I've let them down, myself down . . .* more shame charged in.

Things became a little clearer as I pulled myself together. *I'm doing this for myself, to better myself and be a better person, a greater husband, a greater father and to live a more fruitful and longer life with my family. It's only three weeks. I'll get through it for myself and for them! That's the big picture; that's my motivation.*

I reminded myself of the priceless lessons I hoped to learn there: the coping mechanisms, the control I would regain, all to be able to steer Summer and Joey through their lives. I would be the husband my wife deserves . . . Frankie is the rock in my life, my driver, my love.

After this pep talk, I left my room and was shown around the ward. It was nothing like I imagined, and it was certainly no holiday resort. There were two covered courtyards outside, a meeting room, a kitchen, a small games room with puzzles and cards, a laundry and a dining room. There was no access to the gym or hydro pool unless I was given authorisation by a psychiatrist I was yet to see. My life here would be basically me in my room, alone with my thoughts on how to work on myself, and a schedule of classes and meals.

The first dinnertime soon came, and I made my way to the dining hall. Arriving late, I walked in with my head lowered in shame. I asked a nurse if I could eat alone in my room. 'Sure thing, Michael,' she said. 'The first day is always the hardest, and I understand.'

At 41 years old, I felt like I was going through my first day at school all over again. *I'll push through like I always have. I have to.*

My day ended with my first consultation with the psychiatrist. I told her about my condition, my meds and so on. She quickly assessed and changed my meds. *Maybe,* I thought optimistically, *I've been taking the wrong medications for a while and once they're right, all of my problems will disappear!*

Life in the clinic was built around routine. Each day started at 7 a.m.; soon after I woke up, a nurse would come into my room to take my blood pressure and pulse. Breakfast followed. On my first morning, I was still in pyjamas and slippers when I headed to the dining hall, only to see that everyone else was dressed in normal clothes. I started laughing at myself, and this was my little icebreaker with the group.

A man came up and said, 'You must be a sportsman.'

'Yes,' I replied, a little warily.

'It has to be rugby, right?'

'Yes, how'd you know?'

'I could tell because of all the lumps on your face and scars on your head.'

At 9 a.m. each day, there was a group briefing on the daily program, followed by a meditation session and a range of group discussions. I met all sorts of people there and soon realised that they looked up to me. They nicknamed me the 'BFG', or 'Big Friendly Giant', after the Roald Dahl character. My time in this place didn't just have to be about me: it could also be about helping others who were in need.

A little community, so to speak . . . There's only so much a psychiatrist can do, and I felt that if I could help someone with even one thing, I was doing my job and being the best me I could be. Helping others became part of my daily focus.

Frustratingly, I wasn't allowed to go outside for walks or runs initially, so I got into the routine of an in-room work-out that I designed for myself. It started with seven sets of 25 push-ups and seven sets of 25 sit-ups, and I built it up from there. What more could I do than exercise when I could? After three years of not going to the gym, I wanted to get back into it, hoping for some muscle memory to come back quickly.

My first group session started with personal introductions, in which we described our backgrounds, what caused us to be here and the goals we hoped to achieve once it came time to leave. When it was my turn to speak, I didn't feel any embarrassment. I made myself an open book, which was a relief and a surprise, but I was getting into the spirit of it.

There were a few strong takeaways from that first session in the form of advice from other patients, which included:

- Stay the course.
- Let the information you receive be the tools you'll carry with you for the rest of your life.
- Exercise.
- Occupy your time doing activities with the kids and others close to you.
- Give gratitude and be positive.

- Either change the situation, or change your reaction to the situation.
- Learn to say NO.
- Avoid people or situations that stress you out.
- Control your environment.
- Express your feelings.
- Compromise.
- Create a balanced schedule.
- Adapt the way you communicate.
- Look for the upside.
- Share your feelings rather than bottling them up.

Not a bad first session!

My changed medication regime began to play havoc with me as early as day three. I woke up late, groggy and disorientated, and was late for breakfast. In the dining hall, I rushed around in a fluster and asked the three people lingering in the room, 'Who took my breakfast?'

They didn't know. I stormed into the lounge area. 'Who took my breakfast?'

No one owned up, so I calmed down and asked the nurse for some All-Bran, toast, banana and coffee. Crisis averted. While eating, I reflected on what had just happened. What were the other patients thinking after I basically interrogated them? Knowing I'd overreacted, I went back into the patient living room to apologise. They said, 'That's absolutely fine, it happens a lot around here. It was nothing compared to other events that have occurred.'

I felt reassured, yet still embarrassed. I called Frankie and filled her in.

'You and your food, hey!' she said, and I started laughing. I FaceTimed Joey and got to see him loving life, eating his rockmelon. After I hung up, I didn't get angry or upset, I was just calm. I missed them so much but kept going back to the reasons why I was there.

Even though I was in a clinic that focused on the treatment of addiction, my specific problem was the way my alcohol use interacted with the symptoms of my brain injury. Being off the drink, while it was obviously a good thing in itself, didn't stop a recurrence of these outbreaks of disorientation and panic. The incident with the breakfast was just the first of these. Another time, one afternoon just before dinner, I couldn't find my jumper. This jumper, a present from Frankie, meant a lot to me. I checked under my bed, looked through my wardrobe and took every piece of clothing out to check if it was there, but it was not. I checked the bathroom, behind the curtain, everywhere. My anxiety levels shot through the roof. I headed to reception to see if a navy blue jumper had been handed in by any patients, and the nurses replied in the negative.

Now I was really in a flap. Over dinner, I obsessively gathered my thoughts about where it could be. I retraced my steps over the last few hours, but I just couldn't remember. I finished dinner quickly and headed back to reception to ask the nurses again if anyone had handed it in. Again, they said, 'No.' I went back into my room and turned it upside down looking for my jumper, and lo and behold it was on my pillow!

I was so relieved. I headed to reception, feeling like an idiot, and told the other patients I'd found it. I settled myself, and then FaceTimed Frankie and the family. Trying to describe what I was feeling was difficult; however, it felt like the world had revolved entirely around whether or not I found this jumper. It may not have even been the jumper itself, or the challenge of finding it, or needing to know exactly where I left it. It felt like it was something much deeper than that, involving questions of control and whether I could trust myself to do the simplest things anymore. I shouldn't have made such a big deal about it. It's not like I left the clinic, so it had to be there somewhere. I was left feeling embarrassed and depleted, all over a jumper! I wish things were different.

Another afternoon, just before Frankie arrived to drop off some food, the cursor on my laptop stopped working, and I went into a panic. I repeatedly reset the computer, and it still wouldn't work! *What am I going to do if I can't use my laptop?* I called Frankie. Summer yelled out, 'It must be the num lock button—somewhere up the top of the space bar in the numbers column!' Her solution worked. What a relief, but I couldn't believe what a state I'd got myself into.

'What a legend you are,' I told Summer. 'You'll get a huge present when I'm out of here—thank you!'

Then I accidentally deleted some of the diary I was keeping . . . *Oh my God, I couldn't possibly have done that.*

Isn't it on autosave? I called Frankie again, and she ran me through how to retrieve it. *Thank God for my family! I don't know how to do some of the simplest things in life* . . . I'm not embarrassed or ashamed, I just feel like someone has ripped my ego right out of me. My inability to do simple things, and then my tendency to compound it by panicking and catastrophising, was what I was in here for, as much as the rehab itself. The interaction of alcohol with my brain condition was unique to me—at least at the time I was in the clinic—and I felt that I was fighting on two fronts.

After five days, I was finally allowed outside for a walk. I am not good at sitting indoors by myself, and I was ecstatic when I was given the news. *Woo hoo!* I changed my clothes and got ready for my 5 kilometre walk. *How good!* After being in there for four days, I finally got to go outside and breathe some fresh air on a beautiful 27-degree day, with no wind and not a cloud in the sky. I was champing at the bit . . . *Let's go!*

We were only about a hundred metres out of the clinic when I yelled out, 'The funny farm is coming!' Everyone laughed, and we continued walking. I noticed members of the public looking at us quite strangely, or ignoring us, not saying 'hi' when we greeted them, like they thought we weren't human, when we were just normal people getting out and enjoying a walk like everyone else.

Towards the end, a few patients started to run, so I joined them. The endorphins kicked in, and I felt fantastic! I hadn't been on a run in more than four months due to my severe back pain. So, what made me run now? Well, what's the worst that could happen? I end up in hospital?

Back at the clinic, I was pulled over by one of the nurses who wasn't on the walk/run.

'The nurses were a little freaked out by you!' he said.

'What? How? What did I do?'

'Nothing, other than they couldn't see you after the turning point.'

'But I passed one nurse and said I'm running back to the meeting point.'

'They were still freaked out.'

I was baffled, and my run felt as though it had been spoiled. I'd let someone down yet again, just by running like everyone else. I went to the nurses who were on the walk and asked, 'Were you guys freaked out about me? Why? I mean, this is a self-admitted hospital; I'm not going to run off anywhere, am I?'

They explained the situation: as I was new to the outdoor group activities, they didn't know what I might do. *Ah, okay*. There had been enough times when I didn't know what I might do, either.

In our group sessions, I learned a lot about addiction and how it interacts with a brain injury. I didn't think of myself as an alcohol addict because I didn't drink a huge amount on a daily basis—nowhere near it—but what I learned was that addiction can be defined by patterns of behaviour more than exact quantities. I told the group what triggered me to want a drink. Throughout the years, I'd installed in my brain a rewards mechanism: you need to earn the right to reward yourself. Over the last few years, most—if not all—of my work had been very physically challenging. It's a combination of hard work and a lot of exercise, much like rugby training. On my days off work, I would do as much as I could around the house to earn myself the right to have a drink later on. So, I would work hard and, feeling virtuous, give myself the reward. The morning after, I would feel anything but virtuous. I would say to myself, 'That's not happening tonight.' Then off I would go, working hard again, and history would repeat itself. I felt ashamed and grew annoyed when anyone brought up the topic of my alcohol use, but the teacher told me that this reaction is very normal. I was only defending my system of rewards. What I had to do was change the actual reward so it was something that didn't end up harming myself and those I live with.

During this session, I learned that:

- At least 10 per cent of the population have an addiction to something.
- Around 50 per cent of addiction is related to genetic make-up.
- Around 50 per cent of addicts use the thing they're addicted to as a coping mechanism for the troubles in their lives.

Other life advice I was given included:

- Change the habit, change your routine.
- Have a mini meditation when you feel like having a drink.

- Close your eyes and say to yourself, 'Is this the best decision for me right now?'
- Minimise the triggers that enable drinking.
- Don't hide behind secrets.
- I'm the expert on me, so I should do what works for me, and I will have a positive outcome.
- Either you want a relationship with your family, or your addiction. Make a choice!
- I need to be okay with my sober self.

Everyone was starting to open up, which was great. About a week after I arrived, one of the patients said to me, 'Michael, everyone here has noticed a huge transformation in you.'

'Really? How?'

'When you first stepped in here, you had your head down, clearly not talking to anyone or making conversation, and now you're the life and energy of the group and someone we all really like and want to get to know more.'

Stunned, I thanked them for the feedback. 'I don't really like to open up to many people,' I said, 'but I've realised that we are all in here for the same reason—to better ourselves—so we are in this together. For you to get the best out of me, I need to open up, and for me to try to help you, you all need to open up, too. Thank you.'

Later, the teacher said, 'Addiction is not a spectator sport—eventually the whole family gets to play.'

Hearing that made me quite emotional, as I realised how much I'd hurt my family over the past few years with all of the things they had to put up with. It blew my mind that Frankie had stuck by me. Yes, we'd had fun and some amazing times together as a family, but then I'd let her and the kids down and that crushed me. I should have known better. Now the remorse kicked in. *I don't want to be any more of a burden to them than I already am. I love them, and I'll do this for them and myself.*

As my brain condition worsened over the last few years, I found it increasingly difficult to open up to my friends. In some cases, I was supersensitive to any signs of them turning away from me. Maybe oversensitive. But I also closed myself off, fearful of what I was becoming. While I was in the clinic, on the other hand, I soon got into the habit of dropping my guard for the other patients. They were doing it, too. We were all in this together. To share the deep aspects of your life with a bunch of strangers is admirable. A lot of people out there don't have anyone to talk to, so I considered myself privileged to be able to share my experiences and challenges with these people.

I had some excellent meetings with the psychiatrist. I let her know how the new medication had been helping me, both mentally and physically. I also learned a lot about the way alcohol consumption can badly affect someone with brain trauma. I'm a unique case, she said, so I really need to take care of my body and mind a lot more than the average person. She prescribed an additional medication to assist me with that. I was progressing, and it felt great. As a bonus, she finally cleared me to use the gym and hydro pool . . . You little beauty!

The clinic was a curious mix of long stretches of boredom and a sense that anything could happen at any time. One night, a nurse found one of the patients curled in a ball, crying behind her shower curtain. The next morning, a new patient came in with a dog—an unusual companion in a hospital, but apparently she had nobody else, and her dog really did help with her loneliness. The dog's barking triggered a few complaints, not least from another patient whose contribution to group meetings was to complain about noises that, to my ear, were entirely regular. 'The courtyard door makes a noise when it shuts, so you guys need to fix it!' he would blurt out.

In the middle of my stay, I walked into a group session in which the subject was 'Managing Anxiety', and the teacher said to me, 'You're the mask!'

'What do you mean?' I asked.

In a joking tone, she replied, 'It's someone who puts on a humorous personality to ensure that people like them; however, there's a lot of things going on inside you.'

I didn't know how to take this at first, as the teacher had only met me twice, but I soon realised that she was spot on: I have always wanted people to like me, and that's the personality I carried into the clinic. I don't believe I'm fake. I try to be humorous to ensure that people laugh, have a good time and enjoy my company. But I don't hide anything from the people who matter to me. In the week I'd been there, everyone—including the staff—was getting used to me. 'The life of the party,' they called me. Yeah, right. All we needed was a party.

In that same anxiety session, having disarmed me by seeing my 'mask' so clearly, the teacher got me to open up about my life. The patients seemed interested to hear about my rugby career, how I found the transition into the real world, the person I was now and my life in general. This was confronting for me. I admitted how the transition from playing rugby on the big stage in front of thousands of people to the real world was—and remained nearly a decade later—extremely difficult. 'You go through a self-identity shift,' I said. 'Going from someone whom everyone loved, gave to and did everything for; you had no financial issues; you're playing the game you love with your friends, and you're someone people want to know, be friends with and always want attention from—then it's all gone away in a matter of days.'

Noticing the sad faces around the room, I added, 'Hey guys, it's all good! I have the best wife in the world, who I love more than anything, and two incredible kids who I love to the moon and back. I'd do anything for them; I'd die for them!'

Learning about anxiety made me question my assumption that I didn't suffer from it. Anxiety, we were told, can affect your brain, nerves, skin, muscles and joints, heart, stomach, pancreas, intestines, reproductive system and immune system. When faced with anxiety, people either battle it or remove themselves from the situation (fight or flight). Most people use the flight technique, as they don't like confrontation. A technique that helps with anxiety is to talk to yourself and think about yourself in a positive manner. Don't beat yourself up—life is too short!

We took a ten-minute break. When I got back, the teacher said to me, 'I've just googled you!' Everyone started laughing.

I responded, 'Don't believe everything you read online!'

The teacher, now very intrigued, asked if I could talk to her more later. My small dose of fame, and my history of head trauma, made me a unique patient. Like I say, everyone was different.

One of the most useful sessions I had there was a discussion of dialectical behaviour therapy (DBT), which explores healthy ways to deal with stress and anxiety, and to regulate emotions. We learned the S.T.O.P. skill:

S—Stop and think about the situation you're in that is making you feel anxious or uncomfortable. Do not react straight away because you're not thinking rationally. Simply accept the way you feel. You may think to yourself: *How do I tolerate this?* Don't lose focus by reacting to other people's emotions, as you can't control those. It's not you, so stay in control.

T—Take a step back, breathe deeply and try to relax. You don't want your feelings to make you act impulsively because that won't lead to a positive or productive outcome.

O—Observe what's going on outside and inside you. What's the situation? What are others doing and saying? Check the facts before deciding on what to do.

P—Proceed mindfully! Act with total awareness of what you're doing, to ensure that your actions lead to the best possible outcome for the situation.

One morning while I was still in the clinic, I woke up with a smile on my face because I remembered the last dream I'd had during the previous night. Frankie and I were walking around Bath. We were holding hands, shopping, laughing and dancing in the streets as if no one was around. It was perfect, and we were so in love! Funny thing was, from top to bottom, she was wearing all pink—and Frankie would never wear that! I laughed to myself. This was a nice start to my day, and somehow a reminder that I had turned the corner and would soon be heading home.

I might be deluding myself, but one of the best outcomes of my time in the clinic was that other patients turned to me for counsel and advice. For the first time in years, I was being seen as somebody full of capability and useful experience, and other people were looking up to me.

There was an eighteen-year-old man there, whose experience of being bullied at school was so crippling that it drove him to the edge of suicide. He and I had some long conversations, and he seemed to get a lot out of them. Another young guy was suffering from night terrors that woke me up; after putting my foot in it by asking him who was screaming during the night, I managed to talk him into a state where he was quite calm and almost happy. There was a transgender patient who had been in the clinic for six weeks and was fighting the urge to take their life every single day. I said, 'When you look at yourself in the mirror, do you see a great person, who's kind, smart and funny? Or do you see the person you think people are perceiving you as?'

They said they'd never been asked that before, responded that they weren't sure, and then suddenly said, 'You know what? I am a great person; I am kind, smart and funny.'

We ended up taking in nature together at the beach, watching all the dogs running around like little kids, seeing the eagles flying above as they stalked potential prey, looking at all the people running and the surfers in the water. We ended up running around, too, making jokes, taking the piss out of each other and talking about our families. On the bus ride home I said, 'If you ever need to talk to someone when times are good or bad, I'm here for you and I'm in room ten.' I just hope I gave them a good experience and made them feel better about themselves.

A young woman who was leaving the clinic came up to thank me for my openness and sheer honesty. Suffering from severe anxiety issues and depression, she said that when she was at school, she was bullied frequently due to her weight and, ever since then, she'd had extremely low self-esteem. I was so impressed that she had the courage to step out of her comfort zone and talk to me—it was a step in the right direction.

'You have no reason to be shy, embarrassed or uncomfortable approaching people,' I said. 'You're such a nice lady and are very easy to talk to. I've met a lot of people throughout my life, and you are one of the easiest and most outgoing, intelligent people I've spoken to, even if it's only been for a short time.'

During one of our 9.15 a.m. walks, I opened up to one of the patients about how my parents got divorced when I was eight years old, and I only saw my father every second weekend, as my mum had the lion's share of custody. I didn't really think about it too much at the time because my siblings and I were young, going to school, playing sport and totally naive about the situation. In my mid-thirties, I reached out to my father and we rekindled our relationship. Obviously, we were both struggling with the past, but we pushed through it; now I have my father back, and he has his son back. I'm so happy we have each other again. Frankie played a big part in this, and I thank her every day.

The patient and I agreed that life is short. Be kind, be humble and be happy; love the people you have in your world, be the best person you can be, and try to get the best out of every situation possible. One day, it's all going to be over. We don't know when that will be, so let's live every day as if it were our last.

For the first time in my life, I learned something about mindfulness: be totally present, be purposeful with the task you're doing, and be non-judgemental. It's a great lesson for anybody, but possibly even more important for someone with a condition like mine. The teacher asked, 'Has there ever been a time when you've been totally present and not thought about anything else other than that task?'

I thought back over my past. Funnily enough, rugby never crossed my mind. I said, 'My wife's birthday was coming up, and instead of buying the usual jewellery, flowers, clothes and so on, I wanted to do something different—something heartfelt—which would be both thoughtful and meaningful. My wife used to be a model for Makita, and she was the poster girl for the company, so I decided to draw a picture of her holding a Makita drill, colour it in, then frame it, wrap it and give it to her on her special day. That was one of the very few moments in my life when I couldn't or wouldn't think about anything else other than that. Mainly because it was so important to me to see the elation on her face when she saw the finished product. It was a success and is now hanging in our garage, where a lot of our special mementos are kept.'

Notwithstanding my 'mask', my loss of self-esteem in recent years was one of the primary forces driving me towards alcohol. I didn't understand that I was suffering from a brain injury, so when I felt bad about myself, I sought an easy way to self-medicate. Whatever its manifestation turned out to be, the underlying cause of my bad feeling was a low opinion of myself.

In our self-esteem session, the teacher focused on society's tendency to push us into comparing, criticising and estimating ourselves against some external measuring stick, and then competing against others. Social media has created an easy platform for people to compare themselves to others, which impacts individuals' self-esteem on a daily basis. Even without this, as a sportsman I had been comparing and judging myself against others my whole life. Where had it got me? Yes, I'm competitive and was somewhat successful when I was playing rugby. But it's a hard habit to break, even though there are more important things in life than being better than the next person you are playing a game against. The truth is that I was still judging and comparing when I first walked into that clinic. Why? It didn't get me anywhere, other than on a fast track to feelings of shame, anxiety and regret.

The antidote, the teacher said, was the seemingly simple idea of knowing and being faithful to your true self. If you know your true self, then nothing else matters. Don't compare yourself with some fake concept of others; there's only one you, and you are perfect the way you are.

There are a few ways to get to know your true self:

- Be still and listen to yourself, your heartbeat and your emotions.
- Control your breathing, slow it down, be calm.
- Accept who you are and how you're feeling right now.

Over the course of my life, nobody has known my true self better than my twin brother, James, and one of the highlights of my days in the clinic was reading the emails he sent me. He wrote about how proud he was of what I had achieved throughout my rugby career and also—crucially for me—of the person I had become. He knew my true self, and he loved me. He reminisced about times we had growing up, such as playing basketball against each other on the front driveway until dark, when our mother would yell out, 'Dinner boys, come inside!' We would both run inside, and I would always eat my meal the quickest, and then try to steal food off everyone else's plates. They all called me the 'tin can'!

We were so competitive that there was a war involved in everything we did. James was a fantastic basketball player and a hell of a long-distance runner; I admired his spirit as he did his best in everything, and I looked up to him. Another email mentioned how proud he was of me for coming into this clinic to better myself for my family. I was using the inner drive I was born with for something far more important than stuffing my face or doing well in a football match. These words immediately lifted my spirits and confirmed that I was where I should be. Thanks, James! After this particular email, I was totally re-energised and ready to take on the day.

As much as it cheered me up to be reminded of that part of my history where I was admired, the loss of my rugby career still left me with feelings of grief and loss, which was the title of one of our sessions.

I felt a growing sense of sadness, powerlessness, emptiness and self-pity for having lost the social interaction that alcohol used to facilitate in my life. This spiralled into grief for all the time and money I had lost. It was only when I was in the clinic that I faced up to how prevalent these feelings had been in me.

We went on to discuss the classic stages of grief and loss:

- denial that there's a problem
- anger (the rage inside: 'Why me?')
- bargaining (always finding a way/excuse to have a drink)
- depression (separating the life you once had from drinking)
- acceptance (you accept, learn from and live peacefully with yourself).

Sometimes a solution can be in front of you, but you don't notice it until the time is right. I'd been aware of the classic description of the stages of grief and loss for years, but only now was it ringing true for me personally. I realised that it fitted me to a tee when I came in here . . . every stage of it except the acceptance!

In my final days in the clinic, we began to focus on positive thoughts, particularly relating to self-esteem. We brainstormed what our strengths were. I listed a few of mine:

- disciplined and trustworthy
- mentally strong and hard-working
- highest core family and personal values/morals
- am better with a routine
- know my support network
- honest, loving, caring and generous
- highly protective and reliable
- fun and enthusiastic
- never give up.

Just making that list did me a huge amount of good. I'm not a completely lost cause.

Depression was one of the big topics for all of us in the clinic. As with everything else, we each dealt with it or refused to deal with it in our own unique way. Having seen some of my fellow patients literally at the point where all they wanted to do was end their lives, I could gain some perspective on my own version of depression. I think the clinic helped me both to acknowledge that depression was affecting me and to reassure me that I wasn't in an acute state.

The key takeaway for me from the talks about depression was to determine what is real, rather than to imagine what could be. With my lost jumper, for example, I clearly lost my grip on what was real. I had to teach myself to stop in the middle of that fever and reframe what was occurring.

About twenty minutes into this session about sadness, I started thinking about my family and how much I missed them. I lost it and started to cry. All of a sudden, I got up and left the class. People were asking, 'Michael, are you okay? What's going on?'

I couldn't walk to my room fast enough. Once I was shut in, I let out all of the tears. I called Frankie; she always makes me feel better. I told her, 'I'm not coping . . . I've hit a wall . . . I want to leave . . . I miss you all too much, and I want out!'

Frankie responded sensibly. 'I honestly thought this would happen a lot earlier,' she said, the kindness in her voice very clear over the phone. 'Try to detach yourself from everyone else and their issues, as you're there for a reason. You should stay the course.'

'I don't think I can do it,' I said, weeping. 'It's just draining me—everything is—and it's hit me like a tonne of bricks.'

'Michael, being the life of the party doesn't always have its perks! There's an instant pressure, as people want to be around you, and there's a certain expectation of you. You are braver than most of the people on the planet; because of this, you have the tools you need to get through anything. What you're going through is completely normal. I love you.'

What a woman she is, and how lucky I am.

I gathered my thoughts and headed back into the class, mainly because I didn't want all of the questions from the patients as to why I suddenly left pursuing me for the rest of the day. I apologised: 'Sorry guys, I was just on the phone.'

We moved on to the subject of mood and what lifts it. A few of my mood lifters are:

- exercising as much as possible because it clears my head and puts me in a positive mindset
- being social and interacting with people
- having fun with the kids, whether it is wrestling on the floor, doing puzzles, kicking the soccer ball in the park or playing basketball out the front
- walking on the beach with Frankie (earthing)
- watching sport over the weekend
- working and being active.

To decrease the chance of depression, I learned that I can meditate on and be thankful for everything I have in my life:

- my family and friends
- my life in general (living every day as if it were my last)

- being in this clinic and discovering all I can
- the business I own
- the pets I have
- the roof over my head
- the food I eat
- the happiness my family has together.

This might sound like self-help rhetoric, but hey . . . my 'self' needed a lot of help!

In my final days in the clinic, the nurses finally gave me permission to go for a run on the waterfront. 'Michael, we fully trust you now, so go for your life!'

I felt like a bird being released into the air. *I'm free, I'm free, how good is this?* I ran double the 5 kilometre distance we would usually walk. Pelicans were everywhere. There were families on their boats, guys on their jetskis and other people exercising. I hadn't run for months, but the likelihood of a sore lower back didn't faze me one bit. Back in the gym, I was smashing out daily routines of bench presses, shoulder shrugs, front raises and bicep curls along with sit-ups and push-ups aplenty. I was the fittest I'd been in years. I called my father and had a deep and meaningful chat, as I really needed to tell him a few things . . . and it was great!

When there was a Covid-19 outbreak in the clinic—this was during the Delta wave—things began to change quickly. I saw my psychiatrist, and she gave me her approval to leave five days earlier than my scheduled departure time. There weren't any therapy sessions planned over the weekend, and I was having my second Covid-19 vaccination jab, so I wasn't going to get a lot from the program over those days. I was so happy—I called Frankie straight away to tell her the good news.

In my farewell group sessions, we discussed 'Boundaries' and 'Assertiveness in Recovery'. Both were good for me. 'Boundaries' was important because I had been trained, in rugby, to push myself beyond my limits, and the further I could break my boundaries the better. It was all about setting personal standards or records and then surpassing them. Although this had positive effects in rugby, I saw that carrying the same programmed behaviour into ordinary life could have strongly negative effects. It's good to know your limits because you can self-destruct at any time. We all have our boundaries! People abuse their boundaries due to brain trauma, which made it personal to me: my alcohol addiction was all about applying the same boundary-busting mentality to drinking that I had once applied to sport.

We learned the AAA Principal:

- **Awareness:** being aware of your boundaries.
- **Acceptance:** being able to accept that these are your boundaries and not to cross them.
- **Action:** being able to act, when the time is right, cements your true self.

We then did a little meditation, which I connected with, but things got really weird very quickly. Five minutes into the meditation session, the teacher asked everyone to stand up, open their eyes and start walking slowly around the room (keep in mind that it was a very small room with seven people in it). The teacher then asked us to continue walking and make eye contact with every person, then to shake their hand, then to give them a high five. I felt that this was a very strange technique to use with a group of mental health patients. Most of the patients were extremely uncomfortable, vulnerable and scared. I simply thought it was weird, and I didn't connect with it at all. I understood why the teacher asked us to take part in this exercise, but it just wasn't for me. I left politely, went to my room and called Frankie. She, too, was a little shaken up when I recounted the session to her.

'Assertiveness in Recovery' was better. I have sometimes confused assertiveness with discipline, but they are different beasts. Being assertive means that your needs are met, in a positive way, while you are still respecting other people and not engaging in conflict. When being assertive, you make a statement, for example:

- I must leave here by 4 p.m.
- I am so grateful you're able to come with me.
- I am not too sure about that, so I'll have to think about it.
- I like it when we do it together.

Assertiveness is being firm, direct and honest. You have choices, and make the right one. On the other hand, being passive aggressive includes actions such as:

- feeling one way but doing something else
- being critical of the advice and direction that others give you
- sulking, pouting, dawdling and always being late for things
- being negative and pessimistic
- feeling like you are the victim and having difficulty accepting responsibility
- sabotaging the efforts of others
- feeling envious and resentful of others and subtly antagonistic.

A lot of these points hit home for me. To address them, I had to learn about particular modes of communication. For example, the 'I' message:

- is a direct and clear message describing your feelings
- makes you own your feelings
- tells the other person clearly how you are feeling, without blaming him/her.

On the other hand, the 'You' message:

- is often blaming or judging
- holds the other person responsible for how you're feeling
- causes defensiveness, resentment and resistance.

A great way to start a sentence is:

- I feel . . .
- I would like . . .
- I would prefer it if . . .

This is respectful communication that doesn't produce any further conflict. Needs are met, and everyone is happy with the outcome.

Leading up to my release day, I called Frankie to see if we might all go to the beach to have some quality family fun time, and then go home, have a big rib-eye steak and keep the family fun going with puzzles, basketball, kicking the ball in the park and walking the dogs. She loved the idea; I got excited. I pictured myself walking through the front door and being greeted by my family, all together with uncountable hugs and kisses. The joy of having the kids run up to me is one of the best feelings I can have as a father, and I absolutely cherish those moments, as I know that they won't last forever. The thought of seeing Frankie again was indescribable; she's the love of my life and my best friend.

Even though I was champing at the bit to get out, I really valued this experience. It was life-changing. Before I went into that clinic, I never took the time to actually focus on myself. I was continually seeking distractions, either doing something with friends, playing sport, entertaining or mucking around with the kids. It was great to spend some time working on myself. Not having much scheduled over the weekends, and not much to do after 4 p.m., it was an eye-opener for me to fully come to terms with the person

I was now and where I wanted to be, and to work out how I would get there. I came out of the clinic self-assured in my aim to be the best father possible, the greatest husband to Frankie (who deserves the best of me) and the best friend to those I hold close to my heart. My diagnosis did not have to get in the way of any of that. I was ready!

20

FRANKIE

Adopting Digger

2020–2022

During the Covid-19 lockdowns, people discovered Zoom, baked sourdough bread, kept Dan Murphy's in business and adopted dogs.

I have always owned dogs. Because I was an only child, my pets were my siblings. As an adult, I am that disgusting person who lets them lick me on the face and sleep on our furniture. I don't care—they are part of the family. The only thing that irritates me is the shedding—I have already gone through three Dyson vacuum cleaners! My dream is to one day own lots of land and be able to rescue animals left, right and centre.

We already owned Bob, a little pug–terrier cross named after Bob Hawke because he came into the Lipman residence the weekend that Bob Hawke died in 2019. Michael got to name him because, well . . . I don't actually know why, but for some reason it was his choice, much to Summer's disappointment. Then we noticed that our new neighbours were constantly bringing home foster puppies and rehoming them, and curiosity got the better of me.

'How do you go about fostering?' I asked Trinity, the twelve-year-old future Bindi Irwin.

'We know the people at the rescue centre,' she said. 'I'll pass on your details.'

Soon we were called up, along with our neighbours, to take on some corgi–Jack Russell crosses that had been rescued from a hoarding situation, where one owner had *more than 150 dogs* on the premises. Our neighbours took two, and we took one. The dogs arrived late at night, shaking in their crates, absolutely traumatised, and they clearly lacked experience with any kind of human interaction. We opened the crate and tried to put a lead on one of them, but he bolted away so quickly that none of us could catch him.

What a disaster, we thought. How were the rescue people going to trust us again? We couldn't even get the dog inside the house before he ran away! The poor little thing was MIA on the streets of Davistown. We searched at night with torches, while people in community groups put up 'sightings' on a Facebook page. I assumed that we wouldn't get asked to look after him once he was found. Unexpectedly, I received a call from the rescue-centre person saying that a ten-month-old bull terrier–Arab cross had been surrendered by a country breeder, and asking if we would like to take him instead?

'Only if he is okay with children,' I replied.

'I'll keep him overnight to assess him,' the woman said, 'and I'll let you know.'

At 5 a.m. the next morning, I received a text message: 'He's a big softie—no problems with other dogs or cats and wonderful with kids.'

Great, we thought. *Let's pick up our new foster dog!*

We brought him home. In the animal-fostering system, you put photos and a description of the dog up on a website so people can decide if they want to adopt it. You also name the animal. As it was Anzac Day, we called him Digger. Can you see a theme here? Yes, it was Michael's choice again.

What we *weren't* told was that Digger was petrified of men: tail between his legs, limbs quivering, running under the house type of scared. He was bred to be a 'pig dog' and had failed. He came to us with scars all over his face, having been so badly mistreated. We knew that we couldn't let him go. It was Michael's decision to adopt Digger because Summer in particular had grown so attached to the dog, and he didn't want to break the kids' hearts by sending Digger to another home. However, Digger didn't warm to Michael, and this really saddened and frustrated him.

'Surely, he gets that I'm not going to hurt him by now!' he'd exclaim, after the first week had passed, then the first month . . . and so on.

We had an animal-behaviour specialist visit, which cost us $300. 'He is one of the most traumatised dogs I have ever seen,' she said. 'It could take years for him to come around.'

(Two years on, and Digger still suffers from post-traumatic stress disorder to such an extent that it costs us $250 to get his nails clipped because he must be sedated, even though our vet is female.)

Michael needs instant gratification, so this was not music to his ears. He went from believing that he was doing a wonderful thing for his stepdaughter to thinking he had made a very bad choice that he couldn't retract.

At the start, Michael and Digger brought out the worst in each other. Michael behaved like a five-year-old, declaring, 'If he doesn't like me, I'm not going to like him.' Digger would growl and blow dog raspberries at Michael and then run away whenever he came near.

'You don't understand how hard this is for me,' Michael would complain. He was used to everyone loving him, including dogs.

'You've just got to put in the work, like the trainer said,' I would reply, as encouragingly as I could.

We worked out that Digger would only allow Michael to pat him when Michael was sitting or lying down. This was because it reduced Michael's apparent size and reassured Digger that he wouldn't be belted as he had obviously been before. He would play a game of 'catch', where Michael would throw treats in the air for him. As much as Digger resembles Michael in muscle tone, size and handsomeness, he doesn't have the same paw–eye coordination. His catching is woeful.

At one point, I received a text message from Michael while he was at home, saying that he would give Digger one more month—if things didn't improve, Digger would have to go. It was literally an 'It's me or the dog' text.

How was I going to get through to Michael that Digger did not choose to behave the way he did? His wiring was screwed up. He had gone through so much trauma and was deeply conflicted. It became my mission to make Digger our head-trauma mascot. I had to get Michael to relate to Digger and see the similarities between them. They had both suffered trauma when younger, and it was affecting them now. Michael needed to learn patience, and Digger had to learn to trust. And both needed sedation at times. Once Michael came to understand that Digger was suffering through no fault of his own, but from what he was put through by others—just like Michael himself—the penny dropped. He started to put in the work, and for the first time he showed Digger some empathy.

Michael was the one to suggest that I include Digger in his story. It's a long road ahead for both of them, but they are working on their issues together. I can proudly say that after two long years of digging in his heels and shaking his head violently while trying to wriggle backwards out of his collar, Digger will now comfortably go for walks on the lead with Michael. They make a striking pair.

21

MICHAEL

Concussion Connect

2021

It's a standard weekday afternoon, and I am in the car on my way home. I call Frankie on the phone and ask her if she wants me to pick up food or anything else. It's the right thing to do, to offer to help, but inside I'm begging her: *Please say you don't want anything!* Because I'm pretty sure that whatever she asks for, I'm going to forget it within seconds.

'Thanks, darl,' she says brightly. 'Just eggs and milk.'

With my shoulders slumped and my eyes lowered, I am in the supermarket a little while later, wandering around. I know that Frankie needed something . . . but what? I spend a lot of time searching for clues. I'm too embarrassed to do the obvious: phone her, admit I've forgotten and ask her again.

Finally, something clicks back into place. I remember 'eggs and milk' and manage to find both, as if by some miracle.

But there's always a kicker. I get to the front of the check-out line and find myself facing a self-service machine. I can't remember how to use it. I do something wrong, and the 'Assistance Needed' sign starts flashing above my head, like one of those 'I'm with stupid' signs. A staff member comes over to unscramble for me what is a simple, everyday process for everyone else.

Assistance Needed. It's becoming the theme of my days.

Every day brings a new drama with a new workaround. Frankie and I go to a restaurant, and I get overwhelmed by the menu. I can't take in the number of choices, I can't comprehend all of the words jumping out, and I can't keep any sense of order in my head. So, when it comes to the simple matter of answering the waitperson's question—'What would you like?'—I defer all answers to Frankie. She has to order for two now.

Socially, I am letting fewer and fewer new people into my life because I can't trust myself to act normally with strangers. Recently, I took Joey to a birthday party with his day-care friends. I couldn't make conversation with the other parents. I didn't know if I could trust myself or them. I couldn't open up, or even share the basic details of my life with the adults, so I covered up my awkwardness by paying excessive attention to Joey, running around after him to look after his needs and seem busy. On the inside, I was dying for the whole thing to be over. I dreaded the next time, and I promised myself I would do my utmost to avoid it. I was so scared of forgetting people's names or using the wrong words and embarrassing myself that I avoided conversation with them entirely; by avoiding them, I expected that they would think I was a dickhead, which made me want to double down and avoid them even more. It's bad—I shouldn't be like this, and I wish I wasn't. But I have lost all belief in my ability to do the simplest things in life.

The next night, we drove to Macquarie University in Sydney. It's more than an hour from our home on the Central Coast, and I have been so deeply wedded to punctuality ever since my time as a St Joseph's College boarder, it's almost an article of religious faith for me to arrive on time. I am very rigid about it. Of course, that's a recipe for disaster in Sydney traffic for anyone, let alone someone with my lack of composure. So, the trip was a very fraught one, and when we were a few minutes late, I was sweaty and anxious and my heart rate was way higher than it should have been for such a minor drama.

We were there for a meeting of Concussion Connect, the group that Dr Rowena Mobbs had initiated and I had helped to lead for the previous few months on the Macquarie University campus. Every couple of months, about a dozen of Dr Mobbs's TBI patients and our partners would go there for group meetings. We'd socialise in the foyer with some food before splitting into a patients' group and a partners' group. The patients happened to be all men and the partners all women, but that's just the way it'd turned out—it wasn't a rule.

In separate rooms, we'd sit in a circle and share our experiences. At least one doctor would attend both groups to listen and offer advice. Obviously, the needs of each group are very different from the other. On this particular night, Dr Mobbs was the doctor for my group, and we were discussing aspects of living with TBI and different manifestations of early-onset dementia.

I began the group chat by telling everyone about something that had happened to me that day. I was laying some pavers in front of our garage; it's the type of work I like doing. Since learning how to labour manually over the past couple of years, I have developed a moderate amount of competence. I enjoy the outdoors, and at the end of the day I get a sense of achievement out of finishing a job for the family and actually seeing results.

But that day, it hadn't gone so well. 'I laid a paver, and it was one centimetre out,' I said. 'It doesn't sound like much, but no matter what I did, I couldn't get it right. Just one centimetre—who cares, right? But no, I got obsessed about it. I couldn't control my thinking. I was calling myself all sorts of names, and before long I had totally lost my shit. It was like the end of the world. I couldn't stand back from it and think, *Hey Michael, it's only a centimetre.* It mattered so much to me that it spoiled the whole job, and it spoiled the whole day.'

The men around me nodded. They hadn't been laying pavers that day, but they knew exactly how it felt to lose all sense of proportion, to have that negative voice barking in your ear about how useless you are, then that emotional plunge to the point where that 1 centimetre makes you want to explode.

So that they knew it didn't end in complete catastrophe, I told them what had happened: 'A neighbour of mine, Rob, was driving by. He stopped to see what I was doing and if I needed any help. I *begged* him to stay and help me get through it mentally, to calm me down, to talk to me. He made the world of difference by helping me, just by being there. He calmed me down a lot, and I wouldn't have got the job done without him.'

One of the other men chimed in and said that he couldn't even remember the jobs he'd done around his house that day. He knew that he had done a few things, but because he hadn't written them down, he had no idea. 'This happens in advance, too,' he said. 'If you want me to do any jobs, I tell my wife that she has to write them down. If I'm alone, I have to write them down. But very often I forget to do that, and then nothing gets done.'

The group is a mixture of extremes: obsessive-compulsive disorder, depression and anxiety, anger-management problems, blackouts, amnesia, cognitive failure. What we all have in common is that, for long periods of our lives, we have received repetitive brain injuries.

One of the group, who used to be a high-level boxer, talked about a road-rage episode he had become embroiled in. 'I'm working really hard to avoid these things and not to get involved,' he said. 'But the other driver wanted to confront me. Everything in me was screaming to take him on. But I didn't. I overcame the temptation. Unfortunately, I drove away from the situation so fast that I got pulled over by a highway cop and had to explain myself. Fortunately, they let me off with a warning.' What we knew, from sharing our stories, was that for people suffering what we're going through, every day could seem very, very long, with enough drama to fill a movie.

A recently retired rugby-league player was attending for the first time. The only person in the group younger than me, he told a number of deeply moving stories about his battle with his club to have his situation recognised, and the sense of shame he carried at being designated an 'outsider' for breaking the code of silence around copping head injuries and just getting on with your life. He needed help, and he wanted to help others. He saw himself as the line in the sand that must be drawn for concussion in his football code and was putting everything into winning his legal case and changing his sport for the better.

The group comprises not only sportsmen. A man who used to be a submariner had suffered repetitive brain injuries for years from bumping his head against the walls and ceiling of his submarine as it jolted under the water. Tens of thousands of subconcussions and minor bumps added up to a major brain injury. Another guy, a white-collar worker, had a head injury in an accident, just one injury that left him with possible CTE. He was in the first stage of the illness, like I was a few years earlier, where he suffered from headaches and a sensitivity to light and noise so extreme that he spent whole days in bed trying to cocoon himself in darkness and silence. 'It's hell for my family,' he admitted. 'First I'm just missing from ordinary life for days on end. Then I come out, and I explode at family members because the house isn't as tidy as I like it to be.'

Our meetings are structured so that in the first half we tell stories about our latest dramas or share our problems, and in the second half we hear from the doctors and experts who provide us with information and news, and techniques to deal with our challenges.

During the half-time break, we have a drink and a bite to eat. On this night, I slipped away to go to the toilet. But I stepped through the wrong door and found myself in an elevator. I travelled to the ground floor, wondered what I was doing, came back up to the floor where the meeting was, and then realised that I never made it to the toilet. Just another moment in what Frankie calls the never-ending Michael Show.

The techniques that Dr Mobbs and other experts provide us with, after hearing our stories, are extremely valuable. For dealing with rage, they speak about 'grounding' ourselves. The first thing you have to do is stop. Then you name five things that you can see. You name four things that you can hear. You name three things that you can touch. You name any other sensory experiences that you might be able to have right at that moment. It's a great process, and the next time I lay a paver that is 1 centimetre out of line, I'm going to try it.

Another technique is deep breathing. Slow your breathing to a rate of ten breaths per minute, or one breath every six seconds. We are encouraged to download a phone app called 'Breathe' and to practise deep breathing at least twice a day.

The majority of advice is super practical. I don't think we are capable of taking in much theoretical knowledge, so the practical approach is both easier to take in and simpler to apply. When the guy talks about yelling at his family for not tidying the house, the experts' advice is to set up a system with those family members so they can warn you when they see the signs of an impending explosion. With patients suffering the way we are, there are almost always warning signs leading up to outbreaks. Getting a family member to communicate when they see those signs can be an effective circuit-breaker—but sometimes that's not as straightforward as it seems.

Our experts also import some techniques from cognitive behaviour therapy (CBT). For example, when I and other members of the group get mad at ourselves for doing something like laying a paver 1 centimetre out, we usually abuse ourselves with names such as 'idiot', 'moron', 'stupid' or worse. The experts encourage us to set up a personal 'swear jar' where we reward ourselves for not using those particular words, and for replacing them with something more neutral. Negative self-talk is a real scourge for men suffering TBI, as we have found out during our talks.

When we calm down by stepping back and avoiding the abusive words, it's a great idea, we're told, to go back to little stocktaking lists, such as three things we're grateful for in our life up to this moment, and three things we will be grateful for in this day we are living in. This might sound simple and obvious and straight out of a self-help book. But I can tell you, it works!

I am as proud of my role in starting Concussion Connect as I am of anything else I have done in my life. It started with me seeing Dr Mobbs as my clinician, and her having the idea of bringing patients together in a group, with me leading their conversations. She expanded this idea to the parallel group of patients' partners. When she said that I was the best person to lead the patients' group, as I was the youngest and the most outgoing, I was hugely honoured. When we talk about our symptoms, our experiences and what we're feeling, it's so powerful for everyone—this group is the one place in our entire lives where we know that we will be understood and where nobody will judge us adversely.

We look forward to each meeting. Anyone I know who has any kind of brain condition, I send them to Dr Mobbs, and we encourage them to join Concussion Connect. My ambition is for Concussion Connect to expand out of these small rooms in one venue, using technology to bring us together with a larger community of people who have reached the point of putting up their hand and asking for help. I expect that the great majority of these people will be men, and that involves a challenge to the traditional male mentality. For generations, men have been made to feel weak for admitting to these symptoms, whether they have a diagnosis or not. Change can happen. How do I know this for sure? I managed to change myself.

22

FRANKIE

Empathy Dysfunction

2022

Have we made it sound like after getting the diagnosis, taking the big step to seek help and get off alcohol, and finding a sense of purpose through his involvement with Dr Rowena Mobbs and Concussion Connect, Michael was somehow 'fixed'?

I was really proud of how open Michael was after he came out of Brisbane Waters Private Hospital and appreciative of how much it helped. I think it's such a shame that there is still a stigma surrounding psychiatric treatment. Michael did a brave thing, and we are all better for it.

But you have to remember that it's always going to be a work in progress for us because Michael's condition is not reversible. It is treatable, yes, but that doesn't mean he is always well. A lot of the time, Michael continues to show symptoms of the brain injury he is dealing with every single day.

One of the hardest parts of living with someone who has suffered repetitive head trauma is dealing with their lack of empathy—their inability to see things from another person's perspective, and to feel what they feel. The orbitofrontal cortex is the area of the brain that helps us to react to another person's feelings, so if any part of this brain region is damaged, a lack of empathy can result.

It means that Michael's injuries have made it harder for him to identify the emotions of others. Without knowing what they're doing or how this is changing them, people with a TBI become more self-centred than they used to be. To make it even more challenging for Michael, he suffers from a lack of insight and that can make it hard for him to understand his own behaviour.

Other cognitive and behavioural problems that can accompany a lack of empathy after a brain injury include:

- childish behaviour
- apathy or low motivation
- disinhibition
- aggressive behaviour.

Michael ticks three out of these four boxes! I thank God that I am not dealing with aggressive behaviour. Manic—yes. This is what leads to the arguments, and we have had some whoppers. Normal people would recognise when they've made mistakes and apologise for doing the wrong thing. I am constantly apologising to Michael for things that aren't my fault, just to defuse situations.

Three weeks out of four, I don't bite. I tiptoe around him, smile and nod. Unfortunately, I suffer from severe PMS, which lasts a few days. My hormones are out of control; if there is stress in my life at the time, I am completely overwhelmed, to the point where I feel like I am having a nervous breakdown. If I am poked, I turn into a screaming maniac.

It's the perfect storm, right? In early 2022, I had been working fourteen-hour days dealing with an immense amount of stress in our business. On top of that, all four members of our household—Michael, Summer, Joey and I—came down with Covid-19. Plus, I was very busy writing this book. I couldn't step away from the computer or my phone for a second. I asked Michael, who had recovered from Covid by then, to do some grocery shopping, which he finds really challenging; I also needed him to do a few loads of washing and make dinner. When I asked him to do these things—just to help me out—he took it as a personal attack and pointed out bitterly that he 'was doing everything'. Michael doesn't have a full-time job (he takes on odd jobs here and there), and although it would be great to be in a 'traditional' relationship where I could be the stay-at-home mum and housewife, that's not the way things are.

In the middle of this discussion, it was again clear to me that Michael simply doesn't have the ability to put himself in my shoes. It's an awful position to be in. Michael is an alpha male by his nature and upbringing, and I know that he wants to be the provider, but it's just not a possibility because of his brain disease. We are too proud to ask for government assistance, even though I have been told that Michael is eligible for a disability pension and National Disability Insurance Scheme (NDIS) support. But when he baulks at helping out around the house, it's the straw that breaks this camel's back every time!

The advice is always this: when you are living with a person who is suffering from a TBI, try really hard not to take what they say too personally. Detach. Does that sound easy? Sadly, it is hard to do in reality.

23

MICHAEL

Going Public, Facing the Future

2020–The Present

When I first got my diagnosis, I thought my life was going to be all downhill, on a straight line until I couldn't speak, couldn't remember anything, and would be in a vegetative state needing full-time care. It plunged me into a depression that I addressed, at the time, by increasing my reliance on alcohol.

While I was dealing with the shock and wallowing in my personal pain, Frankie refused to accept that this was going to be the inevitable trajectory of either my own life or ours together as a family. She needed to believe in something more positive, for her sake and for the sake of Summer and Joey. But it wasn't just an act of faith. Through Dr Rowena Mobbs, Frankie was able to investigate the truth about my condition. Getting ahead of me, she discovered that the future need not be a relentless downward spiral. There's a lot we can do to improve our lives and make the decline less steep. There's actually plenty to look forward to. It has taken me some time to really believe this, but now I do.

Frankie and Dr Mobbs faced a challenge to get me to believe in my own future. One of the early steps in that process was to have me accept my condition and drop the mask of play-acting the old Michael, the rugby star, the cheerful fellow whom everybody loved to be with and who cruised through life. They convinced me that a critical step in this acceptance would be to tell the world what I was going through.

In late 2020, Peter FitzSimons came to one of Dr Mobbs's sessions at Macquarie University. Peter was a Wallabies rugby player when I was a kid, and he had since carved out a career as a sportswriter first of all, then a social commentator more broadly on radio and TV, and also as a writer of bestselling books on Australian history. Still a prominent voice in the rugby community, Peter was following the developments of the concussion class action in the NFL and took a typically forthright position on the need for our football codes in Australia to better protect their players from the effects of TBI.

When Peter came to Macquarie University, Dr Mobbs persuaded me to take part in an interview with him. Frankie joined in the interview as well. I was a little bit tongue-tied, worried that I would get my words mixed up in front of an audience, and I struggled with the embarrassment of telling outsiders that I had been diagnosed with early-onset dementia.

Frankie was more forthcoming, telling Peter, 'There were lots of tears. And once we talked about the effects of concussion, and probable CTE, it was like a light went on. We had all of these answers for everything we had been experiencing. Michael had a lot of cognitive tests, and he had a score of seventy-seven out of one hundred, and I thought, *That sounds awesome* . . . I looked it up, and it was really concerning because it was actually at the stage of mild dementia. And I am like, wow, this is what we are dealing with, and Michael's only forty years old.'

Peter also interviewed two Australian sporting icons from an earlier generation, rugby-league legend Steve 'Blocker' Roach and world boxing champion Jeff Fenech. Both told him that they could not count the number of concussions they had suffered while playing their sports, if concussion is defined by having 'white dots in front of your eyes', as Steve put it. What they knew for sure was that there had been hundreds, maybe thousands, of such impacts. They spoke of their own forgetfulness and losing the ability to find words. They mentioned former colleagues in their sports who were now so disabled by confusion and depression that they often could not get out of bed. It wasn't just a few people or the occasional isolated incident: it was virtually an epidemic among retired players of contact sports.

After he interviewed us, Peter contacted Frankie and me and asked for our permission to write about us in the *Sydney Morning Herald*. He said that he would write only the known facts and speak respectfully about me. We said yes; this is our situation, and the sooner people sit up and take notice, the more urgently the sports would be forced to act. Peter also warned us that we would attract scrutiny and even scepticism from defensive sporting bodies and members of the public who were still to be convinced and didn't want the hard physical contact of their games to be whittled away. We repeated to Peter that we would handle that, and in November 2020 he wrote his article. I suddenly went from Michael Lipman, private citizen, to Michael Lipman, one of the best-known cases of an elite Australian sportsman with an early-onset dementia diagnosis resulting from concussion in rugby union.

It's not that I was recognised walking down the street, but when you go as public as I did about an issue that is so sensitive, you become hyper-aware of anyone looking at you. I had been famous, in a small-time way, when I was playing at Bristol and Bath, but this was obviously a very different circumstance. I found that when people did recognise me, they were sympathetic and interested in knowing more. Regardless of whether they were curious spectators of professional sports or parents wondering if they should let their child play rugby, their interest always seemed genuine. In the last two or three years, concussion has gone from the margins to the very centre of the conversation on contact sports.

It wasn't my first time speaking out publicly. Back in 2014, I took part in an instalment of the SBS program *Insight*, hosted by Jenny Brockie, on the subject of kids and concussion. Its focus was on how concussion affects children and teenagers, and it looked at how junior sports might be modified. Studies at that point had found that when kids suffered concussions in sport, a huge proportion were unreported and unexamined by medical professionals, and the kids involved continued to play in the same game (as I used to do) and took no time off afterwards. The protocols fell severely short of adequacy. I appeared on camera to talk about the end of my career after as many as 30 concussions, but Jenny asked me most questions about my ongoing symptoms. I said that I had 'good days and bad days', with headaches and mood swings being the main challenges. I was only a year or so out of rugby. I thought that things were on the brink of getting better for me. How little I knew, and how young and innocent I look in that footage.

Since the article that Peter FitzSimons wrote, I have had literally hundreds of articles written about me or mentioning me as one of the high-profile players in the class action taking place in the United Kingdom. I have come to terms with the exposure and don't feel so embarrassed anymore. With Frankie's encouragement, I have tried to embrace this public spokesperson role as an exercise in leadership. From a young age, I was identified as a leader on the football field and among my peers at St Joseph's College, and for me, ultimately, my public role has helped to rejuvenate my self-esteem.

As much as I like to set an example and talk about what I can do for others, however, my primary focus is on my own and my family's day-to-day existence and wrenching myself away from the pattern of regular dramas and disasters that have ensued from my condition.

As a human being, I have had to rethink my entire role domestically, transforming myself from a traditional alpha male and family provider to a supporter of Frankie and stay-at-home dad for my children. My daily focus is on doing the housework, looking after the kids and being the best person I can be for them. It's all about them now, not me. It took a while after my diagnosis to reconcile myself to this role shift. You have to be brave. I'd already been brave coming out publicly, knowing that being seen as a person diagnosed with dementia would severely damage my employment prospects. But Frankie and Dr Mobbs keep telling me how much I've got to give. My ego has survived. I no longer think that I'm no good to anyone. I have some roles in life that will keep me going. I did lose drive and motivation for a few years there. I lost who I was; more precisely, I lost the ability to adapt to who I was becoming. Now I'm focused on making every day important.

For the first time since I was a teenager, in 2022 I set myself to studying. I enrolled in two courses provided online by the University of Tasmania that are specifically aimed at people who have received an early-onset dementia diagnosis. One of the courses is called 'Understanding Dementia', and the first thing you learn is that if you're diagnosed, there is no inherent limit on your life expectancy. Although I was diagnosed when I was 40, I can hope to live for at least that long again. Dementia is a progressive degenerative disease without a cure, but there are ways to train your brain that will help you lead a happy and productive life. Dementia doesn't have to be your boss. And you'd better get used to it because you might have a very long life ahead of you.

The other course is called 'Understanding Traumatic Brain Injury', and it has been designed to zero in on the particular disease from which I am suffering. When I go out to speak at schools about concussion prevention and what to look out for on and off the sporting field, both of these courses will add a technical understanding to what I can already tell students about the symptoms. They might also help me answer some curly questions!

Another facet of my daily life is helping Frankie with our business. She is the one who does most of the work, but she can't do it alone and I am here to help in any way I can. The major allowance we have to make in that regard is that when Frankie wants me to do things for the company (or, for that matter, the family), I need a specific written list of items and tasks that I can tick off. It has to be simple and precise. I get overwhelmed by too much information, so everything has to be straightforward. It doesn't come naturally to most people, particularly married couples, but we have worked at it. This is something the partners are taught during Concussion Connect meetings.

Dementia, I have learned, varies so much between patients that it's almost a different disease for each and every person. In my case, because I was diagnosed so young, I can make a real difference to my long-term future by changing my diet and lifestyle. If I'm going to live for another 40-plus years, this is essential.

The first thing Dr Mobbs says to anyone with a brain injury is that if they drink alcohol, they should stop. As I have learned, alcohol amplifies dementia symptoms by a hundredfold. Going to Brisbane Waters Private Hospital to get off the drink is the single best thing I have done since my diagnosis. I haven't had to go completely dry: I can enjoy a drink on special occasions. I was never such a serious drinker that I am in danger of falling off the wagon after just one drink. But the key to me stopping my alcohol intake, except for the occasional drink, is awareness. I have to be aware of how alcohol affects me, and I have to listen to what my body and brain are telling me. It's harder for me than for most people, but I can do it.

Eating well is very important to anyone with a TBI. After I went public with my diagnosis, Mark Bakewell, a great friend and past coach of mine, got in touch. He changed my way of thinking by introducing me to the 'Gut to Brain Relationship'. Mark told me how he too, at times, suffered from poor memory, after a long rugby career as an abrasive forward. For the past few years, Mark had only been eating organic products. I'd always eaten pretty well, but Mark took me to the next level. He inspired me to better myself internally and physically through diet. Later, when I studied the 'Understanding Traumatic Brain Injury' course at the University of Tasmania, I learned that between the gut and the brain is an axis that serves as the primary communicator between the central nervous system (CNS) and the microbiome in the gut. The production of neurotransmitters is how the gut speaks to the brain. If you have a TBI, you have an increased risk of getting what's called 'leaky gut', which is an imbalance of the bacteria in the gut which can cause inflammation and irritable bowel syndrome. One result of this is weaker or worse messages to the brain, so your overall movement, speech, breathing, thinking and all the other automatic things the body carries out through daily life is decreased.

As a result of Mark's advice and the study I did, I only drink filtered water (approximately four litres per day), only eat organic meats (mostly chicken or fish, with red meat once a week) and have a balanced diet including proteins alongside vegetables, carbohydrates and fibres. Here is my list of diet basics:

- No soft drinks or fast foods . . . ever!
- Eat pineapple after most meals, as it creates enzymes in my stomach for advanced digestion.
- Limit coffee and caffeine intake. For energy, I use Vitamin B tablets.
- Eat red meat only once a week, only organic or grass fed.
- 'Caught' not farmed fish.
- Vegetables with every meal.
- Two eggs plus one yolk scrambled with baby spinach for breakfast.
- Snacks are mainly nuts, predominantly almonds.

- Limit bread and white rice intake.
- Don't eat too much of anything, as it can cause fatigue.
- Limit dairy foods.

I am very conscious of what I put into my body, as I have to consider every possible option to ensure a longer and healthier cognitive life. A great diet enables me to function better, to exercise more, to improve my relationships and overall enjoy greater wellbeing. I can't thank Mark enough for this!

Just as I have to watch what I am putting into my stomach, I also have to watch what I am putting into my brain, via mental activity. Doing puzzles with Joey, playing card games with Summer, doing crosswords on my own—all of the things that old people are advised to do to keep their brains supple and active—are important for my brain health. The brain is not a fixed entity: it can change and be reshaped by the way you treat it, just like your muscles or your bones. You can keep training your brain to learn new things until the end of your life. Everyone would benefit from doing good daily mental exercise, whatever their age or the state of their brain—but for me, I have had to start doing it earlier than I expected.

Physical exercise is something I understand well and I love. The times I have been unable to exercise, due to injury, have coincided with the darkest mental and emotional periods in my life. I get up early and hit the gym almost every day now. I run if I can, I work out, I swim, I get creative with new routines. Once upon a time, I exercised to get myself into peak physical condition for rugby. Now, I exercise for my own mental survival. The purpose doesn't matter, really; the important thing is to look forward to doing it every day and to enjoy the post-exercise buzz.

When I am out speaking publicly—something I plan to do more and more—everyone listens sympathetically to my story about how I got this condition, and people respect what I say about looking after my family and myself. The lessons about diet, exercise, mental training and quitting alcohol are probably all quite obvious. However, the subject that a lot of people are really interested in hearing my opinion about is children playing rugby and other contact sports. If Joey were to come up to me one day and ask, 'Dad, can I join the local rugby club?', what would I say to him?

That exact scenario is still a few years away, and Frankie will have her own input. Maybe we'll be at odds. Maybe we won't. But for now, I will say that I don't want kids or adults to stop playing contact sports. I don't believe in bans. I don't think they're necessary or practicable.

What I do believe in is safety precautions; they need to be in place and to be strictly observed, without compromise. No whining, 'But it's the grand final next week.' The brain is the brain, and TBI doesn't make allowances for important matches.

There are lots of inconsistencies between sports. For example, in soccer, children under twelve are no longer permitted to head the ball during practice sessions, and if they are between twelve and eighteen years old, they can only practise heading the ball five times a month. In rugby, on the other hand, children of the same age can participate in full-contact tackling. They might be putting their heads in the way of other bodies that are twice their size. While I would not go as far as some experts in recommending that only touch rugby be played before the age of eighteen—and some say tackling should be banned outright—I would like to see more consistent and science-based rules applied across the board.

World Rugby has guidelines on concussion that recognise the fact that children are more susceptible to being knocked out than adults, take longer to recover, can develop more significant memory and mental processing issues, and are more prone to very serious injury from a single heavy concussion. Yet all of the rules in place are about what happens after a head knock. If children show any symptom of concussion, they must:

- be taken out of play and be medically assessed
- not be left alone within 24 hours
- not play again for two weeks
- complete a 'Graduated Return to Play' program involving six steps from a return to normal activity to full-contact practice
- face even stricter tests if they receive a second concussion within twelve months.

All of this is about treating concussions after they occur. None of it is about prevention, other than the tighter enforcement—via penalties and suspensions—of the existing rules. Let's be honest: the only sure means of prevention is to stop all tackling. This is going to be a hot issue in the various sports codes in the near future, as well as between Frankie and me if Joey ever decides that he wants to play rugby. Who knows how we are going to feel at that time, and who knows what rules will be in place? But I can see that if Joey wants to play and I don't want to stand in his way, this is going to be really hard for Frankie.

We are just one family out of millions around the world who will be coming up against this issue of how to look after our children while they play contact sports. I'm not just a disinterested bystander, and I'm no ordinary parent; I want to do something. Dr Mobbs and I plan to develop an easily understood and sustainable program for concussion response in school sports. Once we get a simple procedure rolled out at school level, we can present a more detailed proposal to adult sport, amateur first and then professional. The key parts of this plan are:

- **A limit on full-contact training between matches.** Some teams still practise with full physical contact four times a week. This is ridiculous. It increases the chance of injury and the certainty of repeated subconcussions to the head. There is no reason teams should participate in more than 10–15 minutes a week of full-contact training.
- **Mandatory headgear for under-18s.** I didn't play contact sports until I was eleven or twelve, but I know of kids

playing full-contact rugby league and union from six, seven and eight years of age without headgear. I think anyone whose brain is not fully developed should only play contact sports if they are wearing headgear. Yes, headgear won't stop serious concussions. The back-and-forth rattling of your brain against the inside of your skull will occur from a heavy collision whether you are wearing headgear or not. But the most sophisticated research is finding that it's not only major concussions we should be looking at—it's the number of subconcussions suffered week after week, year after year. In this, headgear can and will help. It just reduces the risk of a multitude of little knocks adding up.

- **Technology.** Mouthguards with microchips are being developed to record how many knocks a footballer is taking. But the mouth might not register a hit to the head. Headgear should also have this technology—then your record of head impacts and collisions for your entire career, including training, could be documented. That would add hugely to the knowledge base for research and could throw up a red flag for the individual, potentially saving their life, if they have exceeded a certain number of heavy knocks in a defined period of time. Covid-19 has shown the many uses of state-based health smartphone apps; I can't see any reason why you couldn't have a regularly updated concussion app that is as useful as your vaccination record.
- **Monitoring.** The technology side is a subset of the bigger issue of having qualified people monitoring all junior

sports for concussions. I have written about the bell-ringer incidents in my career, when I staggered about after a knock, got up and kept on playing, cheered and admired by my teammates and supporters of my club. But beyond those visible episodes, there were hundreds of times when I was at the bottom of a ruck taking huge knocks to the head, either accidentally or from someone intentionally hurting me. By the time the ruck had cleared, I was okay again and kept on playing. This happened at least ten times for every visible major concussion I suffered. And it happens to today's rugby players every day of the week. When it comes to having educated, independent, caring personnel on hand to make sure concussed players come off the field, they must be people who are knowledgeable enough to be looking specifically for concussions in every aspect of play.

- **Education.** Following the previous point, sportspeople must be educated to take matters into their own hands for their own good. Expert observers will not see everything. It's down to the player to self-report. I know that it breaks your heart, now as much as it did in my day, to leave your teammates on the field of play. But everyone needs to be educated so they know that losing a match is nothing compared to losing what I and others have lost through brain trauma.

I love contact sports. I really do. So do millions of spectators and participants. I shudder to think of a future where rugby is possibly banned. I'm even in favour of boxing continuing. Horseracing is another sport where concussions are worryingly common, not only when jockeys fall off a horse but also in the many other situations in which their heads can get knocked around. These sports need to save themselves if they are going to avoid being banned. And they must look after the individuals who have reached a point where their brain injuries have become debilitating.

Do I have any regrets about my rugby career? I do still love the sport, don't get me wrong, but I have regrets about getting up and playing when I was in no fit state, about how long I kept playing when I was concussed, and about playing for clubs and organisations that did not look after me. At the same time, I also regret never quite reaching my full potential. Yes, I played ten times for England. But I wanted to play a hundred times. I wanted to win Six Nations and World Cup tournaments. I never wanted it to end. I mainly just regret being a young man who didn't consider my future and didn't know how much I was putting at risk.

The sports themselves ought to survive, but if they are going to lead to an early death of an individual and a family being put through what I've put my family through, it's not worth it. You've got to pull certain people out of contact sports when their head has taken too many hits. For those unfortunate players, someone needs to step in early in their career and say, 'Sorry, you've had enough.' That's what should have happened during my professional career, and it didn't.

Sport is only the first frontier. The effects of concussion are widespread and worrying in the military services. I have ex-military friends who have exactly the same symptoms as me, due to the repeated head injuries they suffered during their years of training. You don't have to go to war to suffer severe injuries in the military, and the link between TBI and post-traumatic stress disorder in the armed services is only now coming to light. In many areas of manual work, such as the construction industry, landscaping and the trades, repetitive head trauma is a standard feature of the working day. Recreationally, it's cyclists who undergo the most concussions that end up as hospital presentations. The danger of multiple concussions is seen far beyond organised sport.

I'm aiming to take the lead by helping to bring about a positive change to rugby and all contact sports in schools, to club and amateur rugby, to professional organisations, and to areas of the workforce where head injuries occur. If I can speak at a seminar and help twenty people out of a hundred in the room, then I've done my job.

I have a purpose now.

24

FRANKIE

Where to from Here?

2022

There are times I feel so hopeless. Times when I watch my husband sit on the couch in tears—head in his hands because he is frightened about what lies ahead. The sounds of his sobs are unnerving and foreign, like they don't belong in this happy-go-lucky person.

There are moments when I can't understand what he's saying because his sentences are jumping around erratically. When I try to steer the conversation back around, he mutters to himself, 'What am I talking about? I'm making no sense.'

Every night I watch him struggle to fall asleep, then see him struggle to get up the next day. The amount of medication he is on makes my head spin: pills for mood, pills for headaches, pills for sleep, pills for depression. Throw the pills for back pain into the equation, and we could open up our own dispensary.

I have walked outside on more than one occasion to find our car smashed, scraped or run into the neighbour's tree, our tail-lights dangling from the branches like Christmas decorations. *Should he be driving at all?* I think to myself. The lapses in concentration cost us a small fortune in insurance claims.

I have seen the fear in his eyes when he realises that he doesn't recognise someone or can't find the right name for the person he thinks it is in his mind. I have witnessed his embarrassment when he, a grown man, has woken up to wet sheets on the bed because his brain is not sending the right messages to get him up to go to the toilet.

For a time, he drowned his worries in wine, which caused our relationship to suffer so much that we separated briefly, or I kicked him out. I went to Al-Anon meetings, but I knew that he wasn't an alcoholic—he just wasn't coping with the cards he was dealt. I went there to get help for myself when he wasn't yet ready to address the problem.

Some people have taken advantage of his vulnerability in a similar way to how others took advantage of his good nature when he was at the top of his game. I have watched him, broken, coming back from job interview after job interview, unsuccessful and not understanding why. I have sent him out on labouring jobs, knowing full well that it is backbreaking work—the last thing he should be doing after having back surgery—simply because it's the only thing he can do to bring in money to put food on the table.

One day, after telling the world that he had been diagnosed with early-onset dementia, he attended the funeral of a friend who had committed suicide. As he sat quietly at the wake in a bar in Mosman, he was ambushed by a group of men who accused him of trying to destroy the sport of rugby because changes will inevitably be made to protect generations to come. This is a sport to which my husband gave his heart, soul and brain, and he wants to save it now. But some people in the sport do not see this, and treat him badly.

However, through the tough times there is much hope. We are talking about Michael Lipman, a man who can light up a room, who makes everyone feel special, with a smile that wins over the coldest of hearts. He is a big teddy bear, a wonderful father, and in his heart he has a glass filled to the brim with positive attitude. He has been dealt some crappy cards but still has the ability to turn the game around when he puts his mind to it. He took himself off to the clinic to get help, not for himself so much as for us. He is studying at the University of Tasmania's Wicking Dementia Centre, which is not easy for someone who finds it hard to concentrate, in order to better understand what is happening to him so *he can help others*.

I saw how much he could help when, in April 2022, he took the stage to speak at a gala dinner for Dementia Awareness Week. The night was put on by the Bondi2Berry group which raises funds for research towards a cure for dementia. It was black tie, with 330 people in the room, and my heart was in my mouth when Michael went up there with a panel of speakers that also included Dr Rowena Mobbs. We had several friends and family members in attendance, including Michael's father and mother, to support him.

You could have heard a pin drop when he spoke to the room. This was my courageous man. My anxiety turned into overflowing pride as he opened his heart. What an example he set to everyone! The dinner raised more than $70,000, and you could feel the admiration for Michael. He later told me that this would be just the beginning; he has a new purpose to be a game-changer, not only in dementia awareness but in resetting the rules of contact sports to ensure no child starting their career now will end up with the condition Michael has.

Today, concussion protocols in the football codes are being refined and developed at speed. When a top rugby-league player such as Boyd Cordner, the captain of New South Wales and Australia, retires at the age of 29 due to multiple concussions, as happened in 2021, the whole football world gets a wake-up call. It's devastating to us that Michael didn't receive the knowledge while he was playing that concussion and subconcussion were linked to dementia, even though coaches and teammates joked for years about 'how many hits to the head' he had received. He wants to inspire men and women to come forward, seek help and get tested, especially if they have been suffering in silence or confusion or denial. Fans used to cheer for the collisions that would leave him walking sideways, looking at the game with a line splitting his vision in two. It should never be seen as a badge of honour that he played on.

I have a close friend who has made a few mistakes in his time, to say the least, which is why he is serving time in the Long Bay Correctional Complex. Now in his mid-forties, he grew up in Penrith and was as tough as they come, and he used to play rugby league. We chat once or twice a week. A few months ago, he told me about the fits he had been having on and off for a few years. He thought they were from taking human growth hormone, until he realised that they were still happening long after he stopped taking it.

'How many concussions have you had?' I asked him.

'Plenty,' he said. 'I would spew my guts up after every one and feel like I couldn't balance straight for days after. Why?'

'I would put my house on it: those seizures are concussion-related,' I said. 'Are you able to do some tests in there?'

He was able, and did, and the scans came back to show a reduction in cortical perfusion consistent with the suspected diagnosis of chronic traumatic encephalopathy. This is a guy who was diagnosed with ADHD, had explosive bouts of temper but was not an aggressive person, and is looking at a lengthy sentence because of his impaired judgement. I count him as one of my best friends in the world. Like Michael, his concussion history was never linked to any medical issues that arose later on in life. This is my whole point. There is no awareness. A brain is a brain is a brain. An NFL player's brain does not differ from a league or union player's brain, nor does it differ from a military brain that works with explosives, or an epileptic's brain, or the brain of a domestic violence victim. What these brains all have in common is repetitive head trauma. This head trauma causes brain damage. There's no doubt about it.

Mike Adamle, a former NFL player, sums it up best: 'There's something intrinsically wrong with a sport where you lose your marbles.'

Below, I share an open letter to World Rugby's president, Sir Bill Beaumont, published by Progressive Rugby, a non-profit rugby-union lobby group demanding better protection for players. The cost for playing this game that is loved so much should not be dementia. It's too high a price to pay, even if you do get to party with princes every now and then.

Dear Sir Bill,

RE: Brain Trauma in Rugby Union

We write in response to your open letter to the rugby community on 17 December 2020.

This letter is a collaborative effort led by a new alliance of progressive voices in the game under the title 'Progressive Rugby'.

This group includes representatives from all echelons of the game—players, coaches, match officials, club representatives, sports doctors and senior members of the teaching profession.

Both the content and sentiments of your open letter are acknowledged. However, we consider in view of the evidence of risk for traumatic brain injuries occurring in

Rugby Union that more should be done to protect the rugby-playing community from the dangers of injury and that World Rugby has a moral and legal duty to minimise risk and to inform players and parents of the risk of brain damage from repeated knocks.

Evidence of the existence of brain disorders in retired players supports the contention that participation in Rugby Union can cause brain damage. The awareness of the association with traumatic brain injury and participation in Rugby Union is of paramount importance for both the players and the sport itself.

We believe that this issue is the greatest threat to the worldwide game.

Set out below are changes we argue World Rugby should facilitate to our game as a matter of urgency. These are set out in the following categories:

Reducing Injury Risk
Prophylactic Player Welfare
Concussion Management
Post-retirement Welfare
Access for All

This list is not exhaustive, but more a launching pad towards a safer, more sustainable game. Where appropriate, we have prepared preliminary costings for these proposed changes to show that we are sensitive to the practicalities involved.

1. Reducing Injury Risk
   Training:
   Limit on contact in training
   Games:
   The ruck to be refereed as set down in the laws of the game
   Straight put in at the scrum
   Tackle area:
   Review of 'double teaming' tackles; tackles; upper level of tackle height; timely release of ball following the tackle
   Limiting substitutes for injury only
   Workload:
   Careful control of workload in training
   Limit on the number of annual international matches for players

2. Prophylactic Player Welfare
   Career health 'passport' for players
   Health MOTs [Measurements, Observations, and Tests] pre-season and at end of career (to be included in 'passports')
   Central World Rugby Concussion database for incorporation in 'passports'
   Increased education at all levels of head injuries and concussion management

3. Concussion Management
   Research:
   To always include an independent 'broad church' of experts to appraise current research, risks and protocols
   Training:
   Training-ground protocols and access to experienced assessment should be equivalent to game time
   Protocols:
   Extension of the minimum number of days before 'Return to Play' to at least three weeks
   Mandatory comprehensive screening as in other sports after recurrent concussions
   Personnel:
   Review of minimal clinical experience (additional to educational courses) to be present pitch side

4. Post-retirement Welfare
   Concussion Fund to be established by World Rugby
   Ownership of player 'passport' (see above)
   Establishing a more empathetic relationship with insurers

5. Access for All
   Each national Union to be responsible for developing databases of medical specialists able to provide appropriate assessment and advice post-concussion (Public and Private Practice)
   Training packages to teach safe tackling techniques for young players

We firmly support the core physicality that comes with an 80-minute game of rugby union and understand that the game cannot be turned back to a 'rose-tinted' memory of the pre-professional game. Our backing extends to maintaining tackling in schoolboy rugby. However, the above proposed changes are essential to ensure the survival of the game in terms of long-term player welfare and playing numbers at all levels.

While we acknowledge the importance of continuing well-constructed longitudinal prospective research, the rapidly accumulating anecdotal evidence has reached a point that the answer is to err on the side of caution. The alternative is to 'kick the can down the road' for future generations of administrators to deliberate upon.

The NFL has metamorphosed from a sport in denial to a proactive organisation with initiatives like concussion funding and changing protocols to the game, such as the regulation of contact in training, concussion spotters and a concussion tent at each game.

Despite the current negativity surrounding the game, there is an opportunity for rugby to turn the page and follow the example of our American cousins. The current and future generations of players require urgent action to be assured that they will be adequately protected and cared for.

As a next step, we request a chance to speak—as teammates, not as opponents—with senior figures at World Rugby to discuss how we can work together to get control of this issue that threatens the very future of our game.

Michael is not alone in his diagnosis, and there are plenty of people he can help. According to the latest figures, of the half a million Australians who have been diagnosed with dementia, just under 6 per cent, or 28,300 people, are aged in their early fifties or younger. A Dutch study has estimated that 3.9 million people worldwide have early-onset dementia. Although the cause is not always traumatic brain injury, these people suffer symptoms similar to Michael's—from saying the wrong words to becoming disorientated—and they need the right tools to help them through the rest of their lives.

Michael is finding his purpose. He is dedicated to working alongside Dr Rowena Mobbs and promoting her vision to change concussion protocols in sport right down to the grass-roots level, and he helps in clinical and research strategies.

Michael will be a catalyst for change.

25

MICHAEL

What Matters Most

When I think about what matters most to me, I always come back to my family. Deep down, I only really care about the people who are close to me. It's strange to say this, but I don't harbour any great ambitions for myself. My time is done. I have had to put limits on my personal goals, and now, after years of struggle, I can say that I'm fine with this. I want to be part of the backup staff for others now.

I don't know if I will live for another five, ten, twenty or forty years. None of us does. In my case, I also don't know how my dementia will progress in the years I have left. The hardest thing for me—what really brings tears to my eyes—is picturing the day when I have to tell Summer and Joey that I have a brain injury which may lead to Alzheimer's disease or even early death. How do you say that to your children? How do you say it to yourself?

Am I going to be a constant burden on my family? Are their roles in life going to change in order to make allowances for me? Will Summer or Joey have to give up travelling the world or chasing love or having adventures in some faraway place because I am in a healthcare facility and they don't want to leave me? Will I be restricting my children's employment prospects? I'm so scared of putting that on them. It's probably the worst demon facing me; it scares me shitless, the idea that I will be a burden on them when they are still young. When I'm 47, Joey will be nine. What kind of father will that nine-year-old boy have in five years? It terrifies me. I can't put it any other way. It terrifies me every single day.

But in the last couple of years, I have at least improved my trajectory. I have been made aware of what I can do to better myself. I've been educating myself, and if you're not educated you don't stand a chance.

I did not want to write a book. When Frankie first suggested it to me, my embarrassment came to the fore. I didn't want a single person to know about my diagnosis, so why should I put it on paper and tell the whole world? But I changed my mind because I know that my story can help others. That's my purpose now: to give you something to take away from my story that might save your life.

26

FRANKIE

The Fire Pit

We live in a two-storey white-weatherboard house with a Colorbond roof. It is surrounded by timber decking and timber fencing; we don't have a backyard per se. Our house is unique in our neighbourhood in that it is set well back from the road, with a swimming pool in the front.

Michael loves sitting around a fire, which is great when you have a big, open backyard with no fire hazards close to the flames, a properly functioning sense of balance to ensure that you don't fall into the fire, and a memory good enough to ensure that you put the fire out when you are finished with it. This is not our situation at all!

One day while Michael was labouring on a construction site, he met a guy who made steel fire pits that he personalised for his customers. Not long after this, Michael came home with a very beautiful and sweet gift for the family:

a rectangular fire pit with our names cut out of the steel on each side.

As he carried it through the door and proudly presented it to us, I felt my panic rising. 'Oh, that's nice,' I said, trying my very best to be positive. But I was sure that my pained smile spoke the truth. I was terrified. 'Where will we put it?' I asked.

'Out the back,' Michael replied.

As I mentioned, we have no backyard. This meant that he was going to place the fire pit on our wooden deck, which—needless to say—is a dangerous place for it. Obviously, the best location for a fire pit is far from any flammable materials. Within a 1 metre radius of the spot Michael had chosen on the wooden deck, we had a wooden fence, wooden staircase, trees and a trampoline. This is without even considering the fact that the heat and sparks could damage the deck itself and set fire to it.

'I don't think that's ideal,' I said, hastening to add: 'I'm not trying to be negative, but the house could go up in flames.'

But he could think of nowhere else to put it. 'Jesus, Frankie, can you just be thankful and grateful for the gift?' he replied. 'I've done something nice for the family. The kids can toast marshmallows!'

Despite, or because of, Michael's keenness and need for approval, I started to cry. 'I think it's beautiful, Michael. Please don't make me seem ungrateful; I just know what you're like, and the risk is too great! I don't want us all to be burned to the ground in our sleep.'

What should have been a really happy moment soon turned into an argument.

Michael, being as stubborn as he is, didn't budge, insisting that the fire pit was going on the deck.

I replied, 'You're going to at least need to put tiles or something under it.' In case the message wasn't getting through, I exclaimed, 'You CANNOT have it on a wooden deck!'

Michael won. The fires started getting lit, and he would sit by the fire pit for hours. The rest of us tentatively toasted marshmallows a few times, but the novelty soon wore off. I would go to bed, leaving Michael still sitting resolutely by the fire, as if he could make his wishes come true by staying there. His willpower is tremendous, and I love him for it, but this time it was like he was willing into reality something that could only really exist in his head.

Late at night, he would come inside. 'Is the fire out?' I would ask nervously.

'YES—stop nagging me!'

But I knew that the fire would not be out. He thought it was out, he wished it to be out, but I couldn't rely on him getting up at the end of his vigil—when he had been sitting there wishing we were all with him in the way he had pictured when he ordered the fire pit—and keeping in his mind the responsibility to make sure it was no longer burning.

I would wait until he was asleep, walk outside and pour buckets of water on the fire. It got to the point where I just couldn't let him have a fire if I wasn't home. Was that controlling? Probably. Did I trust his memory? Absolutely not.

One evening, I was woken by a massive thump. Michael had fallen down the five stairs from the upper balcony to the lower deck and landed right by the fire pit. It was not uncommon for me to wake up in the morning to find blood on our sheets and Michael having no recollection of how he had injured himself the night before. His spatial awareness, which is not the best at any time, is particularly restricted at night. Watching him walk in the dark is like watching someone walk on the moon. Even on a flat surface, he can grope for each step like he is going down the stairs, arms out in front, trying to work out where he is. It's really confronting for a young and athletic man. Having got used to it, I now just steer him in the direction he's trying to go.

Unfamiliar surroundings are the worst. One time he locked himself out of a serviced apartment in his underwear, while trying to find the toilet. He slept in the hallway; at 5 a.m. he found a passer-by on the street and borrowed their phone to call the after-hours service to let him back into the room. These mishaps can seem quite comical—sleeping in the neighbour's car (as Michael mentioned in Chapter 6) or in a hotel hallway in your underwear—but they aren't funny when you know that the reason for them is early-onset dementia.

The good news? Our fire pit is still out the back, and occasionally we will use it to cook a South African *potjiekos* (stew). I have come halfway to meeting Michael's wish for this little family space around the fire pit that has our names on it. Michael has also come halfway, realising that if he can leave gas on in a kitchen for two hours and not recognise the smell, then having a fire pit running every night with only himself to supervise it is probably not the best idea anymore. He'll go to his best mate Tim's farm and sit around his fire pit for as many hours as he likes. And that's perfectly fine with me!

ACKNOWLEDGEMENTS

MICHAEL

Thanks to:

- My friends and family, who have continually checked in on me and shown their support.
- Dr Rowena Mobbs and her team, for their continued treatment and care throughout my journey of head trauma.
- The team at Brisbane Waters Private Hospital, for their amazing treatment throughout my time there.
- The team at Red Light Rising in the UK, for sending me a red light, which assists me on a daily basis.
- A special mention to Malcolm Knox, for the person he is and openly accepting me to tell my story to him. The way he describes me, my life and my brain condition is truly amazing! Not having our regular chats on a daily basis will feel like I've lost a friend. It's very rare for me to open up to anyone, let alone someone who, at first, was a stranger to me. I've accepted that it's part of his profession, however he is now implanted in my heart and someone I admire and deeply respect.
- Tom Gilliatt, Tom Bailey-Smith and the team at Allen & Unwin for publishing this book and being incredibly supportive and easy to work with.

- Lastly to my wife, Frances ... Our path together has thrown its ups and downs, however in the years to come, your path may be totally different from mine and this is what scares me the most. In twenty years, who knows where my brain will be? It might still be working in a stable condition; I might be lost and not know who you or our kids are! My time may have passed and now my brain is being studied, where will it be? Will you be the one looking after me, or someone else? I might not know, I truly hope I do, however 'the unknown' is the only thing that scares me and consumes me every day. Always know and remember that I love you, Summer and Joey, more than anything in the world!

FRANKIE

Firstly I would like to thank Peter FitzSimons. You might seem like an intimidating alpha, but you are one of the most genuine people I have ever met, full of empathy and compassion: a journalist who showed so much care that you let us read your *Sydney Morning Herald* article before you broke the news about Michael's diagnosis of early onset dementia and probable CTE. I will always be grateful to you for treating our story with grace and understanding, and for constantly checking up on us along the way. This book was your idea.

Malcolm Knox. I don't know if anyone else could have voiced Michael as well as you did. You helped me convince my husband that this book was his biggest act of bravery yet. A legacy rather than an embarrassment. We decided on a 'warts and all' approach for the greater good and I am so thankful for the sensitivity in your storytelling. You must be the most patient man on earth and a true genius to help us piece together timelines and events. Thank you for your belief in my writing ability, your advice and guidance.

Dr Rowena Mobbs. We are so lucky to have found you. I hope this book brings much needed awareness to your mission to understand CTE and younger onset dementia. Thank you for your patience, for being my lifeline. For listening and asking what my needs were when we first spoke in 2020. I suggested that a support group for partners could help and it grew into Concussion Connect. Thank you for helping me understand what was happening inside Michael's brain; I truly believe you saved his life. You are stuck with us forever!

Denise Imwold—Mum, thank you for your unwavering support. You take the kids without complaint when we have to work or attend doctors' appointments or when I needed extra time to get those final chapters in without a three-year-old pulling on my leg. You have listened without judgement, witnessed our battles and quietly taken our daughter off to swimming carnivals, and driven thousands of kilometres up and down the freeway each week to ease the workload of a shared-custody arrangement. You have never asked for anything in return. Thank you for instilling my love of reading and writing, and your continued encouragement.

Thanks to the friends and family who reached out from the time we found out about Michael's diagnosis, to his time in the clinic and beyond. Your offers of help and your genuine care will never be forgotten.

Alix and Mel Popham—for understanding more than anyone what we are going through. We are here for you and love you both.

Whilst writing this book I had two unexpected pregnancies on the pill which resulted in two miscarriages. I want to thank my girlfriends who always checked in to see how I was going, wiped away my tears, gave heartfelt advice and warm hugs. Lots of the time I appear like I have it all together when inside I am a crumbling mess. You are the friends in my life who have seen the good, the bad and the ugly and have remained my rocks. You know who you are and I am forever grateful.

Thanks to our talented art teachers at Pinot & Picasso Hunter Valley. You are the backbone of our business and have made it into the success it is today. We couldn't do it without you!

To Michael, Summer and Joey . . . you make my world a better place to live in. I love you.

INDEX

INDEX

INDEX

INDEX

INDEX

INDEX

INDEX

INDEX

INDEX

The Australian CTE Biobank

The Australian CTE Biobank is the first biobank in Australia to study those with traumatic encephalopathy syndrome and risk of chronic traumatic encephalopathy (CTE).

Their aim is to address the gap in awareness and research for those with CTE, as well as related conditions such as concussion, post-concussion syndrome, and post-traumatic headache.

By observing the trajectory of these patients, they hope to better understand ways to improve clinical care and service delivery for greater quality and quantity of life.

The Australian CTE Biobank's goal is the prevention, care and eventual cure of CTE.

For more information visit www.ctebiobank.org